THE BOOK OF
BABY
MASSAGE

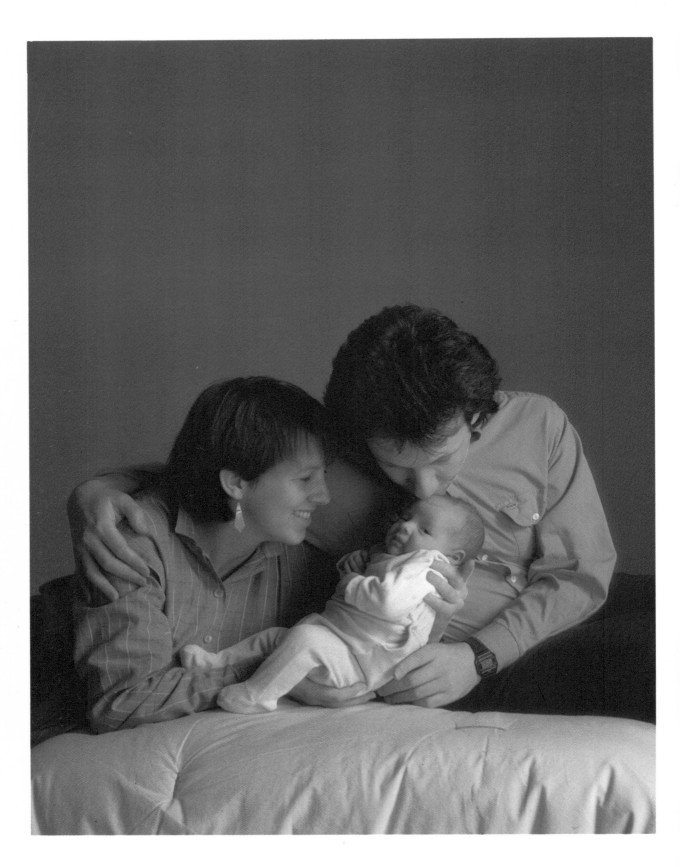

THE BOOK OF
BABY
MASSAGE

For a happier, healthier child

Peter Walker

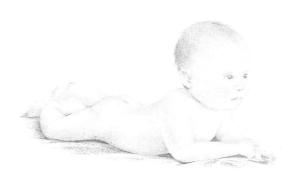

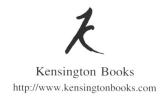

Kensington Books
http://www.kensingtonbooks.com

A GAIA ORIGINAL

Written by Peter Walker

Photography by Fausto Dorelli

Project editor:	Susan McKeever
Design:	Sara Mathews
	Kate Poole
	Margaret Sadler
Illustration:	Sandra Wood
Production:	Susan Walby
Direction:	Lucy Lidell
	Patrick Nugent
	Joss Pearson

KENSINGTON BOOKS are published by

Kensington Publishing Corp.
850 Third Avenue
New York, NY 10022

ISBN 1-57566-282-5

First published in Great Britain in 1988 by Bloomsbury Publishing Ltd.

First Kensington Trade Paperback Printing: April, 1998
10 9 8 7 6 5 4 3 2 1

Printed in Spain by Mateu Cromo Artes Gráficas, S.A. Madrid

ABOUT THIS BOOK

The Book of Baby Massage is a book for both mothers and fathers, a book to improve trust and confidence, and develop a better understanding of your baby.

The book is in three parts. Part One deals with what you need to know before you begin to massage your baby and shows you the easiest and most comfortable way to proceed.

Part Two provides instruction for massage sequences and routines, and shows how, depending on your inclination or your baby's mood, you can either massage one part of the body or complete a whole body routine. These sequences and routines start from birth onward and each one is clearly outlined to suit the different phases of development.

Part Three illustrates the stages of development from sitting upright to walking and shows how best to assist your baby to achieve his or her natural motor skills.

Massage has a wide range of benefits for your baby. Not only does it provide the means to stimulate and relax the soft tissues of the body, it also allows you quickly to recognize any areas of consistent or acute discomfort or stiffness in your baby's body. If you do notice an area of particular sensitivity, do not hesitate to consult your physician for reassurance and a professional diagnosis.

Lastly and most importantly, massage is not meant to be a mechanical routine. It should only be practised with the full co-operation of your baby, and this is obtained through love, affection, and lots of kisses and embraces. Above all, baby massage is intended to be a playful therapeutic activity that will bring pleasure to both you and your baby.

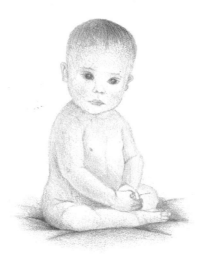

CONTENTS

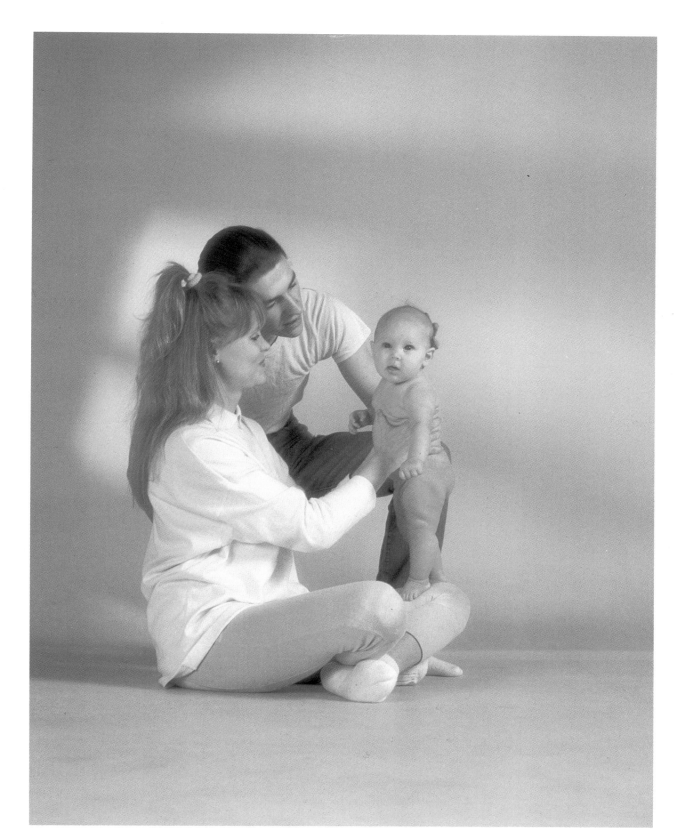

FOREWORD
by Janet Balaskas

More than ten years ago, my two youngest children, who were babies at the time, had the great good fortune to spend many hours in the company of Peter Walker. Even in those days, before his own children were born, Peter had a most unusual and very special attraction for babies. Somehow, as soon as he entered the room, their little faces would light up with joy, all whining would instantly cease and the fun would begin! I could be assured of a break of an hour or two, knowing that I would find them contented and happy when I returned. I tried to analyse what he had that I hadn't, and finally had to admit that despite the fact that he was not a mother (and not even a parent yet), Peter had a natural knack with babies. The secret lay in the way he communicated with them. He spoke to them simply and directly, and related to them with a warm and effortless physicality which let them know instantly that they were in safe hands. Peter understood babies. Above all, I observed, the key to his success lay in the way he played with them. Unlike most of our friends, who held them tentatively and seemed a little afraid of them, Peter communicated directly and spontaneously through touch. Although in those days, he didn't massage them intentionally, I noticed he would often rub a tummy or stroke calmly down the back or hold them in a position that would allow the neck and spine to extend freely or encourage the natural flexibility of the hip joints.

My children loved it. In the hours he spent with them, Peter taught them to enjoy the pleasure of their bodies, to gently extend their physical potential in a way that enhanced their natural development. He helped me to realize that ease of physical communication between parents and their babies is of primary importance and that often the reason that babies cry is simply out of boredom or lack of physical contact and exercise. As my confidence in handling my children grew I noticed how few people were, like Peter, "in touch" with babies.

Touching and physical play are skills which are partly learned and partly instinctive. The learning which might come naturally in a more traditional society, where even young children are used to handling babies, is often sadly lacking in our modern world. All too often we are out of touch with our selves, each other and our own instincts.

In my work with pregnant women and their partners I aim to help them discover their instinctive potential for giving birth naturally and nurturing their babies. Alongside this work, Peter has developed a system of massage and exercise which helps mothers and fathers to enjoy an easy and loving physical relationship with their babies in the months and years after the birth.

I am honoured to be asked to write a foreword to this delightful book which is guaranteed to add so many hours of joy to family life and to enhance and enrich the pleasures of infancy and early parent-hood. *The Book of Baby Massage* is clearly and sensitively written and is easy to follow. Without any complicated techniques, it guides parents to discover their intuitive skills in handling their baby with the confidence that comes from understanding his or her developmental potential. The simple wisdom contained in its pages will help parents to be in touch with their baby from the very beginning, to comfort, soothe or ease minor ailments, and to form a loving and trusting relationship for the years to come.

Janet Balaskas

Janet Balaskas, founder of The Active Birth Movement

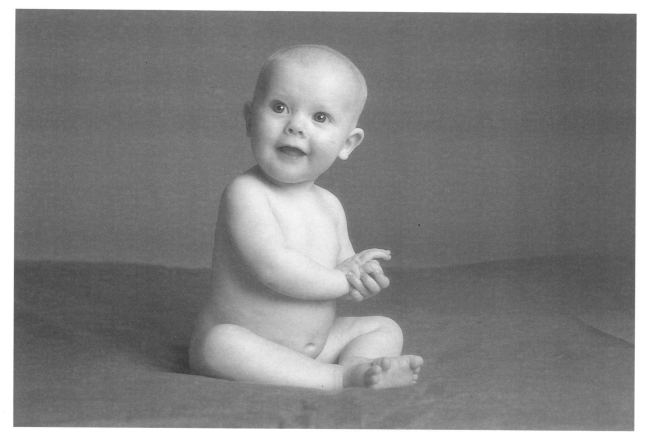

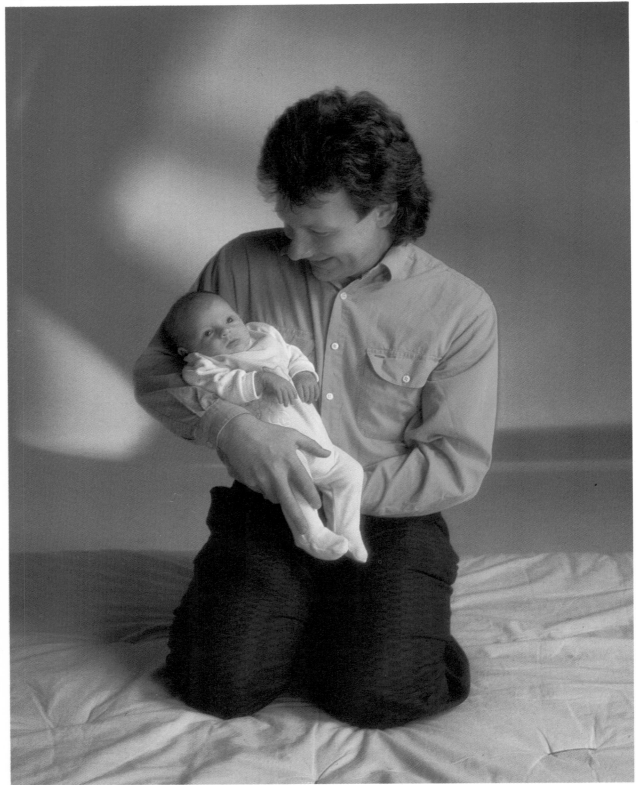

Introduction

Rocked, cradled and nourished in the warmth of the mother's womb, the unborn baby becomes naturally accustomed to a constant embrace and to the immediate fulfilment of all his or her needs. Birth interrupts this secure state and from then on the baby is completely dependent on the love and affection of his or her parents to make the transition from the womb to the world with the least amount of anxiety.

A sense of touch

Touch is the first sense to develop. It is also the baby's most predominant means of communication. All babies respond to the way in which they are touched and handled, and taking the time necessary to get the "feel" of their baby is the most obvious way for parents to get to know their child. Most new mothers and fathers make initial contact with their baby tentatively, touching only with their fingertips. Then, as their confidence grows, they progress to feeling and stroking the baby with the whole hand.

As adults, a lot of what we think and feel is expressed through our hands. Trust and confidence are conveyed by holding and touching in a firm but relaxed manner, while insecurity and anxiety, by contrast, can be conveyed through rigid arms and inflexible grip. Parents who develop their sense of touch and cultivate close physical contact with their child generate ease in their relationship right from the start, and are able to soothe their child with far less difficulty. They remain, literally, "in touch" with their child and this encourages security, confidence, and independence and reflects in the child's personality and in his or her relationships with others.

Both the way in which parents hold and touch their children and the frequency with which they do it are known to have a considerable effect on the child's general disposition. Observation has shown that children who are deprived of physical contact generally suffer more from anxiety and its related disorders. They are inclined to be clumsy in their physical relationships with their peers and, as adults, may find difficulty in responding to others. By contrast, more loving secure personalities are seen to emerge from families and cultures who touch and embrace one another frequently as an expression of their love and friendship. Although, of course, all parents hold and touch their children, many do it only in a very general sense and few parents consciously acquaint themselves fully with their child's physique through their sense of touch. Even fewer parents develop this sense to include massage.

The value of massage

Massage is the original art of "rubbing better", of creating ease through any and all parts of the body. It is an extended form of touch which, developed with guidance and practice, will give you a greater knowledge and understanding of your child. Massage is a constructive, nurturing response to your baby's inherent need for physical contact, one that provides your baby with distinct advantages and ensures that he or she remains relaxed and fluid in movement.

During the early months of life babies uncurl from their foetal position and as they do so they stretch their muscles, open their joints and co-ordinate their movements. Massage is especially suited to these formative months as it provides a cohesive force that encourages muscular co-ordination and suppleness and helps prepare the baby to perform co-ordinated physical skills and activities.

Massage for mobility and health

At no other time in life is massage likely to be of more benefit or so well received as when the baby is preparing his or her body for upright postures and mobility, and needs sustained physical contact. Practising massage during these early months is made even easier because the child is content to remain in one position for a reasonable period of time. From Africa to India, from the South Seas to the Arctic, massage plays an integral part in baby care. From the ancient Greeks and Romans to today's athletes, sportsmen and women and physical therapists the world over recognize the benefits of massage and include it as a valuable means of preparing the body for activity and improving mobility and relaxation.

Massage stimulates the circulatory and immune systems and benefits the heart rate, breathing, and digestion. It provides a perfect balance and support to the development of the baby as he or she co-ordinates and strengthens. It also cultivates the resilient elastic quality of the muscles and improves their ability to relax both in action and at rest. Massaging your baby regularly will give you the opportunity to keep a check and discover any areas of the body that consistently give rise to discomfort, pain or tension. With a toddler, a knowledge of massage can be invaluable as it presents an immediate and effective means to treat and relieve the effects of the minor bumps and knocks that he or she inevitably suffers when striving to achieve balance.

This book gives step-by-step instruction and comprehensive massage routines, endeavouring, in each routine, to show the easiest way to obtain your baby's full co-operation. As babies, infants, and children alike respond best to activities which give them pleasure, each sequence and technique explained in this book is intended to be practised with love and affection. Without this they will simply become mechanical routines. With a little patience and perseverance, these techniques will add mutual trust and co-operation to your relationship with your child and extend your dimensions of play. Daytime and night-time, pacifiers, comfort blankets, and cuddly toys have their uses, but they make poor substitutes if your baby needs the warmth of human contact and companionship. Practised regularly, you will find that baby massage will become intuitive and will help fulfil your child's need for contact as well as providing many benefits to his or her physical and emotional health and development.

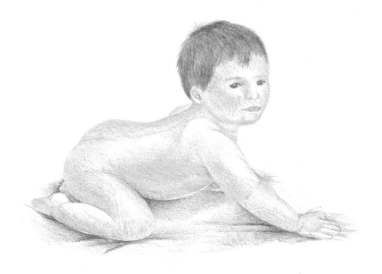

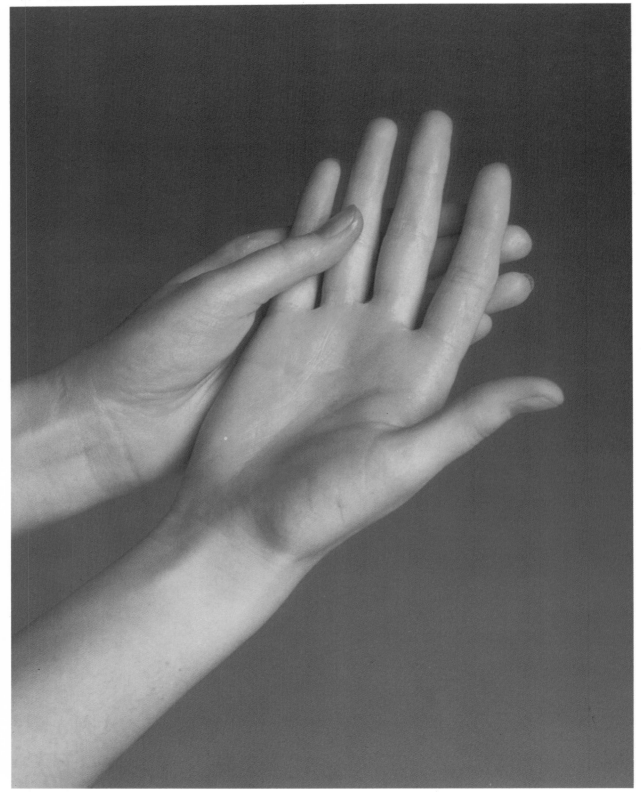

1
PREPARING TO MASSAGE

To ensure that your baby gains maximum benefit from his or her massage, a little prior thought and preparation are needed to maintain your baby's comfort and receptivity throughout.

The best time to start massaging your baby is between feeds, when your baby feels neither full nor empty. As muscles react to the cold by contracting, your baby will be unable to relax if he or she feels at all cold. Babies lose their body heat about ten times faster than adults so check that your room is warm enough and will remain so for the duration of the massage. Also, have a soft comfortable surface ready for your baby to lie on, such as a folded blanket covered with a towel, but don't lay your baby on wool as the combination of massage oil and wool can cause a skin reaction. Keep a supply of clean diapers and a soft towel within easy reach in case they are needed. Also, make sure that you yourself are comfortable and can remain undisturbed for about thirty minutes.

Before beginning, put your massage oil in front of you. Check your hands are relaxed and warm and that your fingernails do not overlap your fingers. If you are using an oil for the first time, check that your baby is not allergic to it by rubbing a little on to an exposed part of your baby's skin and leaving it there for about thirty minutes to test for a reaction. So that you don't have to break contact during the massage, always pour some oil into an open bowl or container so that you can easily dip in the fingers of one hand while your other hand maintains contact with your baby. Use enough oil for your hands to glide comfortably over your baby's body, and make sure you warm it first by rubbing your hands together. Never pour oil directly on to your baby's skin.

Do not attempt to massage your baby against his or her will. If your baby does not react in the way that you anticipate, a little gentle perseverance may help, but if he or she is clearly uncomfortable, stop and try again later. Your baby may be feeling poorly.

Lastly, massage is meant to give mutual pleasure, so don't let yourself become distracted, and keep your attention on your hands. If massaging your baby feels pleasurable to you it is all the more likely to be the same for your child.

MASSAGE OILS

Only the purest oils and the most subtle aromas are recommended for baby massage, because of the sensitivity of both your baby's skin and your baby's sense of smell. First, check that the oil you buy has been "cold pressed", as this indicates a very pure form of distillation. As basic massage oils that do not sit on the skin's surface and block its pores, grapeseed, coconut, and sweet almond are among the most suitable. They are all light and easily absorbed, and coconut is also obtainable in a solid form, which avoids the consequences of spillage. Grapeseed is practically odourless and makes a good base for the dilution of the highly concentrated oils, known as essential oils. All these oils are comparatively inexpensive and widely available from drugstores, supermarkets, and health food stores. Apricot kernel oil is less common and more expensive, but it is particularly good as a basic massage oil for those with extra-sensitive skins and delicate complexions. As an aid to your baby's recovery from some minor ailments, a few drops of an essential oil can be added to your basic massage oil, when appropriate (see pp. 90-92).

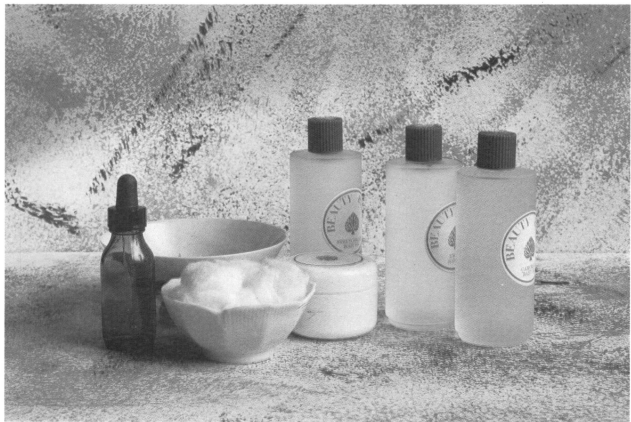

POSITIONS FOR GIVING MASSAGE

Before you begin to massage your baby, make sure that you are relaxed and comfortable. With a little practice you will be able to maintain the same position for twenty minutes or so, but meanwhile change position if necessary. There is no point in putting up with discomfort while massaging as this will make you feel ill at ease and your baby will sense it and also become uncomfortable. Balanced postures and relaxation go together in massage, so whenever possible, try to sit in a position that allows you to lean forward from your hips and lift your buttocks, rather than bending your back. A great deal of strength resides in the back muscles, and once your back begins to bend continuously, these muscles weaken, and debilitate your body's energy. Whenever you can, try to keep your back straight, but not in a "chest out, tummy in" fashion, as this takes far too much effort. As the natural flow of strength is down the back, it can be held straight quite comfortably by pulling down from your shoulder blades and letting these muscles straighten you when you feel your back rounding.

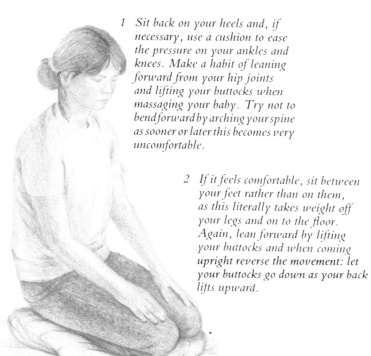

1 *Sit back on your heels and, if necessary, use a cushion to ease the pressure on your ankles and knees. Make a habit of leaning forward from your hip joints and lifting your buttocks when massaging your baby. Try not to bend forward by arching your spine as sooner or later this becomes very uncomfortable.*

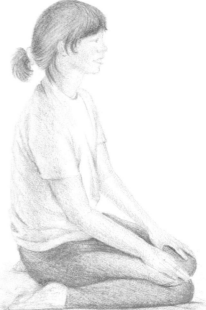

2 *If it feels comfortable, sit between your feet rather than on them, as this literally takes weight off your legs and on to the floor. Again, lean forward by lifting your buttocks and when coming upright reverse the movement: let your buttocks go down as your back lifts upward.*

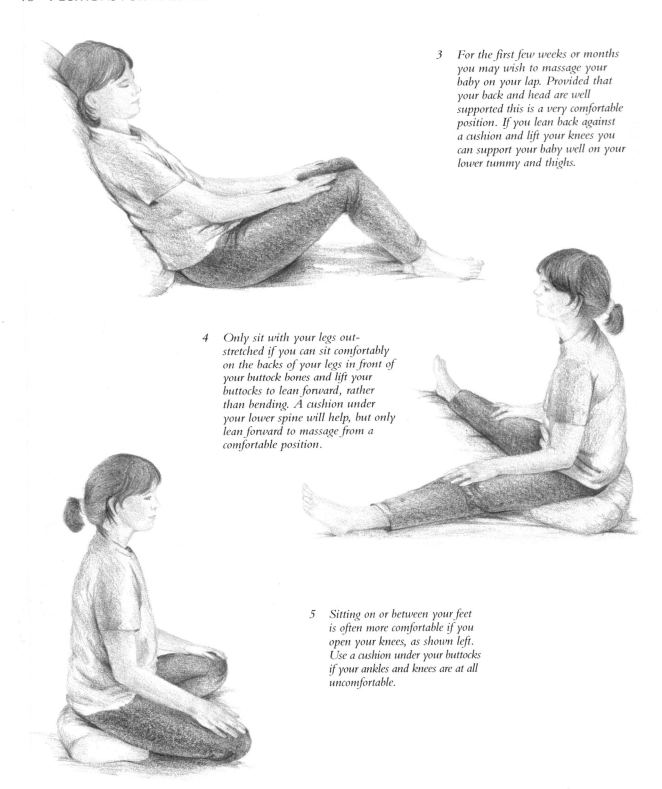

3 For the first few weeks or months
you may wish to massage your
baby on your lap. Provided that
your back and head are well
supported this is a very comfortable
position. If you lean back against
a cushion and lift your knees you
can support your baby well on your
lower tummy and thighs.

4 Only sit with your legs outstretched if you can sit comfortably
on the backs of your legs in front of
your buttock bones and lift your
buttocks to lean forward, rather
than bending. A cushion under
your lower spine will help, but only
lean forward to massage from a
comfortable position.

5 Sitting on or between your feet
is often more comfortable if you
open your knees, as shown left.
Use a cushion under your buttocks
if your ankles and knees are at all
uncomfortable.

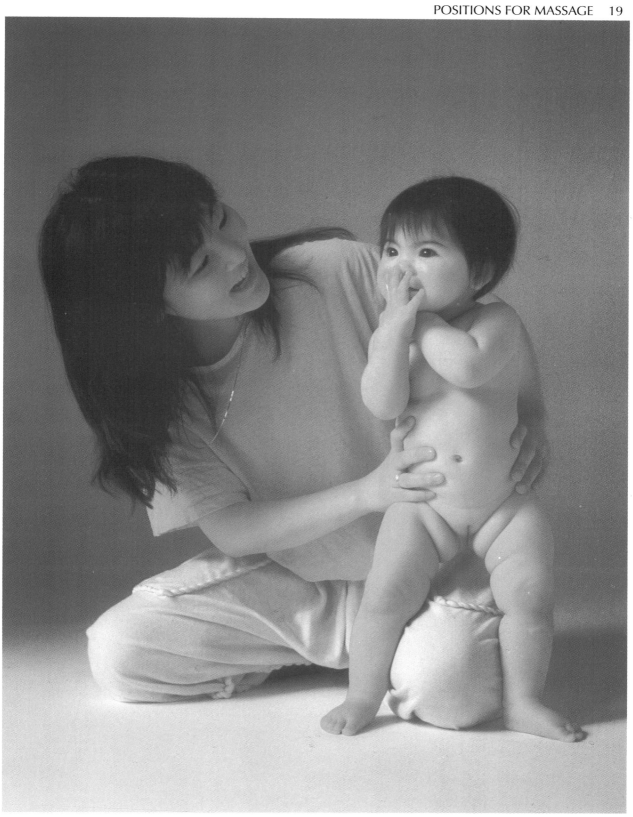

RELAXATION

Sitting properly and maintaining a conscious level of relaxation in action can easily become a useful habit, conserving your energy and keeping you more emotionally centred and stable. Before you begin to massage or handle your baby, check to see whether you are acting under stress, or whether you are relaxed. Two areas of your body that particularly reflect its emotional state are your tummy and your neck and shoulders. These areas are influenced by, and can in turn influence, your inner state of ease and well-being. As an emotional centre your tummy is affected by your breathing and when you are under stress, as your breathing gets shallower, your tummy tends to tighten with anxiety. Check therefore that your chest and tummy are working together – that they expand and contract in unison with every in- and out-breath. If they do not, gently tighten your tummy on the exhalation to push the air out and relax your tummy on the inhalation and allow it to expand with your chest. Check also that your neck and shoulders are relaxed, for during times of stress the shoulders are inclined to lift, to protect the very vulnerable neck and throat area.

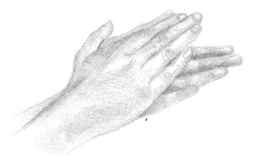

1 Before you begin to massage your baby, sit comfortably, pour a little oil on to your hands and, keeping your fingers straight, rub them together fairly rapidly until you feel the palms of your hands becoming warm.

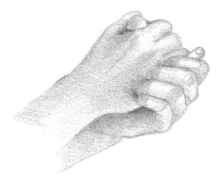

2 Now encircle both hands with your fingers and "wring" them one over the other, clockwise and anticlockwise, until you feel the backs of your hands becoming warm. Now open your fingers, interlock them and rub them together.

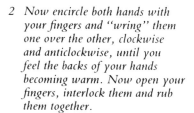

3 Relax your shoulders, lift your hands, and gently shake them from the wrists for about twenty seconds. Now "wring" them again for about the same length of time.

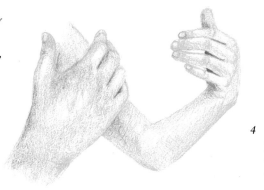

4 To test the quality of relaxation in your hands, lift your forearms and allow your hands to go limp. They should feel warm and relaxed.

5 Encircle both forearms simultaneously, one hand on each, and rub them backward and forward several times from your wrists to your elbows. Now cross your arms and rub the backs of your upper arms until they feel warm.

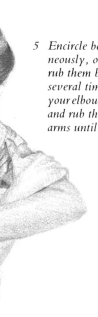

6 Gently massage the tops of your shoulders with your fingertips, then uncross your arms and massage your neck and the back of your shoulders. Now let your shoulders, arms, and hands relax and breathe from your tummy.

MASSAGE TECHNIQUES

From your baby's response, you can discover the pressures and rhythm of touch that he or she enjoys the most. Generally, the very young baby needs to be held securely and, when being massaged, touched gently and slowly. As your baby develops, he or she may well respond more to a slightly firmer touch and a faster rhythm. But every baby is different, and the touch and rhythm he or she prefers may even vary from day to day, according to mood and disposition. In the routines given in this book the direction of massage strokes remains the same, in order to complement the various functions of the body. For tummy massage, the clockwise direction of movement is the same as the digestive rhythm and the movement of food through the large intestine. Massaging the chest, the upward and outward movement of your hands follows the action of the upper ribcage during inhalation. You massage the back downward, in the same direction as it develops strength, and the same direction that its muscles pull to lift the trunk upright. And for the limbs, the downward direction of massage is intended to encourage the arms to open and the legs to straighten, naturally and in keeping with your baby's development.

1   *Start by using fingertip pressure, as this is often the kind of touch the very young baby responds to best. Having already relaxed your hands as shown previously, fingertip pressure is maintained by keeping your hands relaxed from your wrists and keeping light contact with the pads of your fingertips.*

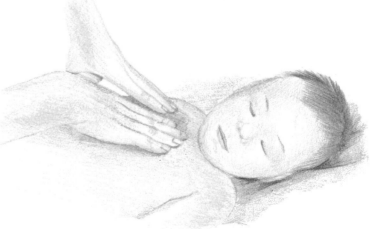

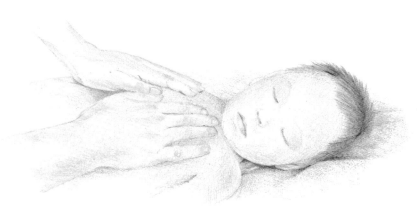

2   If you feel that your baby will
    respond well to more pressure, use
    your whole hand and maintain
    contact with your palms and
    fingers. Again, make sure that
    your hands are relaxed from your
    wrists and use only the relaxed
    weight of your hands, without
    exerting force.

3   When encircling the body's
    contours, like the shoulders or
    limbs, feel the shape evenly with
    your whole hand, using both your
    palms and your fingers.

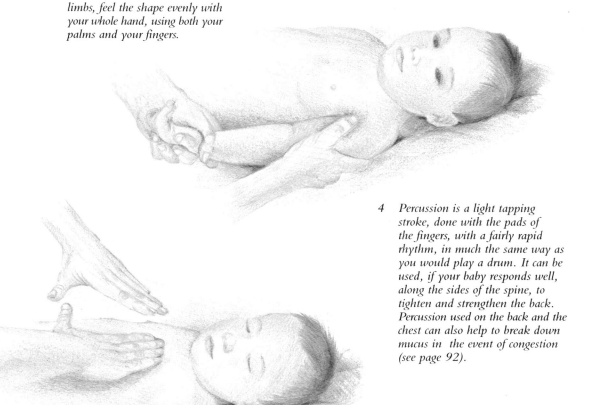

4   Percussion is a light tapping
    stroke, done with the pads of
    the fingers, with a fairly rapid
    rhythm, in much the same way as
    you would play a drum. It can be
    used, if your baby responds well,
    along the sides of the spine, to
    tighten and strengthen the back.
    Percussion used on the back and the
    chest can also help to break down
    mucus in the event of congestion
    (see page 92).

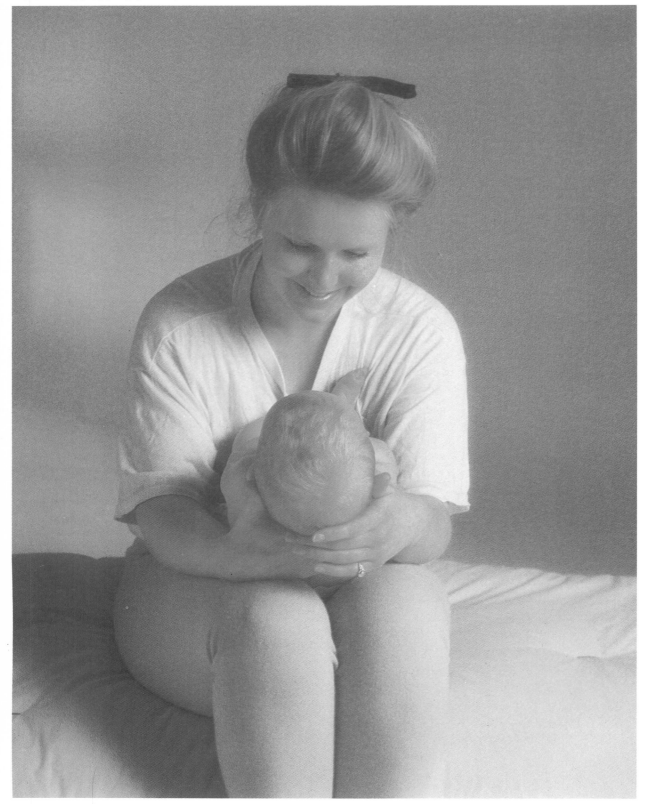

2
MASSAGE ROUTINES

The techniques and routines presented in this chapter will provide you and your partner with the simplest means of transforming your touch into massage. They are designed to give you a starting point from which you can develop your own unique approach, guided by your intuition and your baby's responses. From stroking and feeling the contours of the baby's body during the later months of pregnancy the techniques shown progress to a series of caresses for the newborn, massage routines for the very young baby, and for the young baby from three months onward.

As touch is a tangible expression of affection so massage is nourishment, and during the early months massage is made all the easier as the child is extremely receptive to physical contact and more involved in muscular co-ordination than in mobile activities. Practised at this time, a little regular massage will improve your understanding of your baby and help him or her prepare for later activities. Sitting, crawling, standing and walking are all developed skills and the following routines encourage co-ordination and the even development of strength and suppleness that your baby needs to achieve these skills. From the very beginning, these techniques are meant to be complemented by other expressions of affection. Without love, massage, like any other activity, becomes dull and mechanical and your baby will quickly withdraw. Talking, singing, kissing, tickling and looking into your baby's eyes will all increase the pleasure and benefits of this period of communication.

Although these routines are in no way intended to substitute for medical care you can use them to relieve some of the minor ailments that may affect your baby and soothe the knocks and bumps that inevitably accompany the trials and errors of infancy and growing up. If your baby does not respond well from the beginning, check that he or she is not uncomfortable, cold, or hungry. If your baby shows consistent signs of discomfort in specific areas, check with your doctor or pediatrician. Practised with love and sensitivity, the following routines will add a new dimension to the relationship both you and your partner share with your baby.

MASSAGE IN PREGNANCY

During pregnancy many women intuitively stroke and massage their abdomens – especially in the later months when the mother-to-be often soothes her unborn child during moments of disquiet. In the late stages of pregnancy you may feel the baby's head and back, buttocks, arms and legs as they push at various times against the protective wall of the abdomen. Around this time you may also see and feel your unborn baby's response to external sounds as he or she may jump at the slamming of a door, become noticeably active in response to loud upbeat music, or acquiescent in response to more soothing sounds. During the quieter moments of pregnancy, try stroking your baby through your abdomen. Given that your baby responds to sound as well as touch, playing some relaxing music can help to create more favourable conditions for you both. Using a pure oil, like wheatgerm, will also enhance the massage and can help maintain the elasticity and tone of your skin.

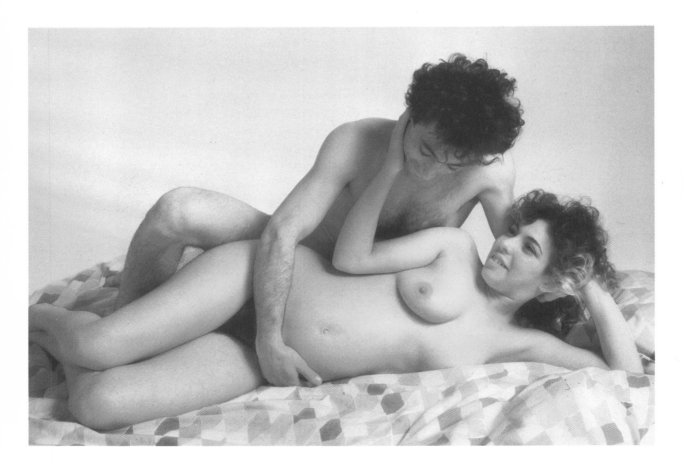

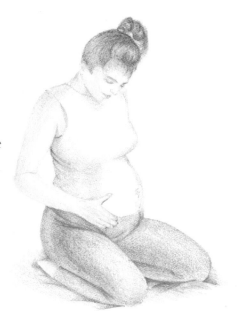

1   Sit back on your heels, placing
    a cushion under them if this is
    more comfortable. Or sit with
    your upper back supported against
    something solid, like a wall.
    Gently stroke your tummy, feeling
    the contours of your baby's body.

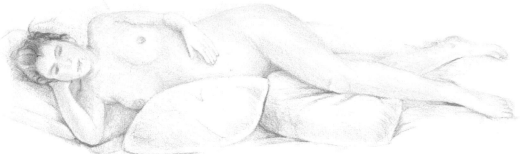

2   Lying on your side, well
    supported, is another position in
    which you can stroke your unborn
    child. Place a cushion under your
    tummy and one under your knee.
    Be sure to stroke gently, as
    your baby may well kick or
    become active in response to a
    firm touch.

3   If you feel your baby enjoys this
    gentle massage, you may also wish
    to share it with your partner. Not
    only will this acquaint him with
    the unborn baby, it will also
    increase the closeness between you.
    You can position yourselves as
    shown right, or in whatever way
    feels comfortable for you both.

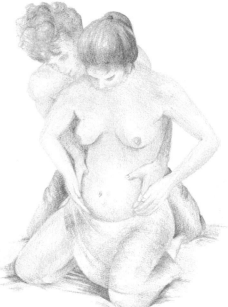

THE NEWBORN

Stroking is a natural expression of affection, and in the same way that mammals stimulate their young by licking them, most mothers intuitively stroke their newborn babies. Stroking is a soft, non–intrusive introduction to massage and you can practise it with your baby clothed, whenever and wherever you are together. Though it is usually confined to the baby's head and back, stroking can just as easily include your baby's arms, legs, chest and tummy. As a new father, holding and soothing your young baby may not feel easy at first, and many new fathers continue to feel "out of touch" with their babies through lack of experience. So be sure to take an active part right from the start. Your baby will enjoy being held and stroked and will eventually come to anticipate it. The ideal time to introduce a massage routine is when you have all got accustomed to the "feel" of one another. Be attentive to your baby's response and begin by spending a few minutes on one part of the body and, when confident, slowly include the rest of the body.

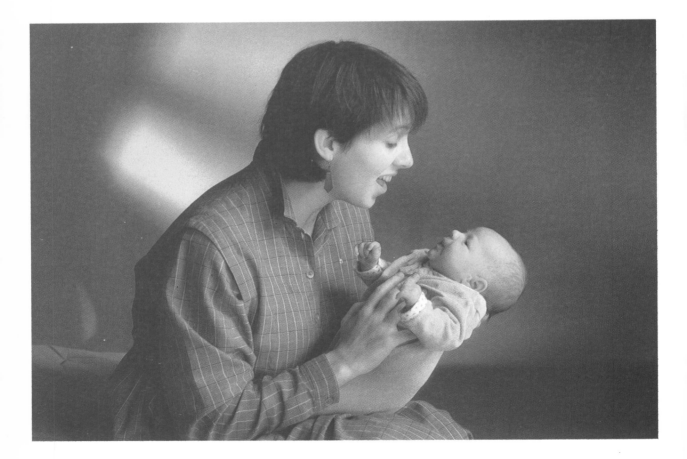

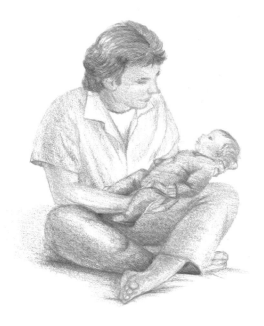

1 Sitting comfortably, hold your
baby in both hands, with one hand
supporting the lower back and
buttocks and the other supporting
the upper back and head. Slowly
and gently "bounce" your baby
by lifting and lowering your arms
and hands. Keep your movements
smooth and look into your
baby's eyes.

2 Rest your baby in the crook of one
leg with his or her legs open and
astride your other leg. Cushion
and support the head with one
hand, and stroke the top of the
head softly in a clockwise direction
with your other hand. If your baby
resists, leave it and try again later.
If not, gently feel the shape of your
baby's head.

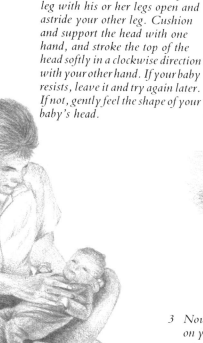

3 Now place your free hand lightly
on your baby's chest. Stroke with
your fingertips in a clockwise
direction all around the chest
and gently feel the front and
sides of your baby's ribcage. Rock
your baby by gently lifting and
lowering your leg and keep talking
to him or her.

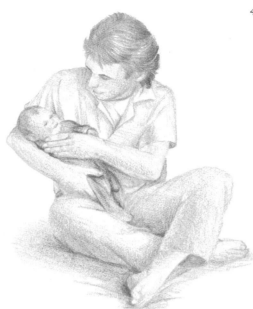

4 Gently lift your baby and settle him or her in the crook of your arm, supporting the head with your upper arm and the back and buttocks with your forearm and hand. Place your free hand over the shoulder and upper arm and squeeze and stroke lightly along it. Maintaining eye contact, gently feel your baby's shoulder and arm. Continue for as long as your baby enjoys it.

5 Now rock your baby by gently lifting and lowering your arm, keeping the movement smooth. Place your free hand around your baby's forearm and squeeze and stroke it lightly, but do not try to straighten it. Repeat movements 4 and 5 on the other arm, but stop if your baby becomes discontented and continue again later.

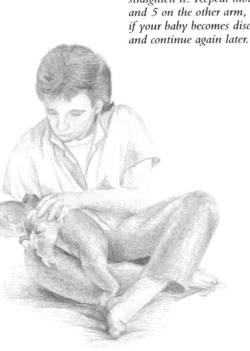

6 Gently lay your baby down face forward, leaning over one of your forearms, hands, and thighs. Place your free hand on your baby's upper back and stroke lightly around it in a clockwise direction. At the same time, rock your baby gently by lifting and lowering your leg. Gently feel your baby's upper spine and ribcage and shoulders. Continue talking to your baby and engaging his or her attention.

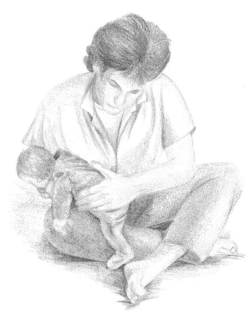

7   In the same position, rock your
    baby slowly up and down and
    place your free hand around your
    baby's side. Stroke lightly in a
    clockwise direction and get the feel
    of where your baby's lower spine
    connects with his or her hips, the
    "wings" of the hips, and the soft
    side walls of the tummy. Leave the
    front of the tummy until the navel
    has healed.

8   Now place your free hand across
    your baby's buttocks, and rock
    him or her gently from side to
    side. Stroke lightly in a clockwise
    direction and gently feel the base
    of the spine, and the buttocks.
    If your baby shows any signs
    of restlessness, stop and continue
    again later.

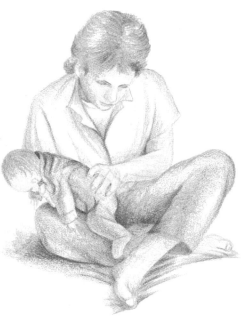

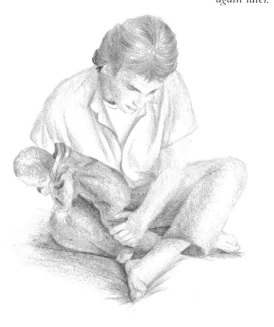

9   Place your free hand around your
    baby's leg and squeeze and stroke
    lightly from the thigh to the foot,
    but don't try to straighten the leg.
    Transfer your baby to lie over your
    other thigh, and repeat this, and
    movements 6, 7, and 8, on your
    baby's other side, keeping his or
    her interest engaged.

MASSAGE SEQUENCES

As you may not always have the time to complete a whole body massage routine, the following sequences are specially created for specific areas of the body. Most of the sequences provide massage techniques both for young babies and for those over three months. The sequences are ideal for spontaneous massage of those parts of the body that are easily accessible – during bathtimes, for instance, diaper changes, or simply during the times that you spend sitting companionably with your baby. As the young baby wants and needs as much close, affectionate physical contact as possible, the positions given allow for maximum bodily contact with your child at all times. As soon as your baby has started strengthening, you may find that he or she enjoys backbending and stretching. For those that do, include the positions that allow the baby to stretch backward over your lap, leaving the front of the body more open for massage.

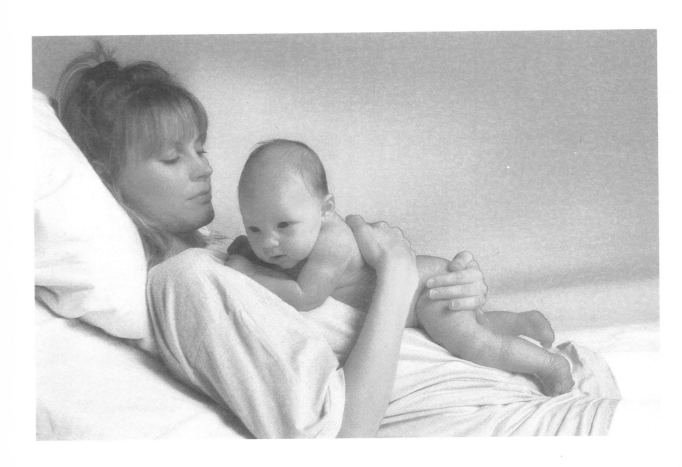

CHEST AND SHOULDER MASSAGE

To be able to breathe with an easy, natural rhythm, the chest and shoulders need to be completely open and relaxed. The chest consists of a complex framework, the ribcage, which supports and protects the heart and lungs, and comprises the breastbone and twelve pairs of bones which are attached to the upper spine. The ribcage has 108 joints which are steadied by a great many muscles. It is the elastic quality of these muscles and the flexibility of the joints which allow for full use of the lungs and free circulation in the enclosed blood vessels. Regularly massaging your baby's chest and shoulders encourages this flexibility, as well as opening and relaxing the front of the body. Although from birth, your baby naturally adopts the best possible breathing rhythm of inhaling and exhaling only through the nostrils and breathing into the abdomen, this rhythm may change if the airways get blocked or the chest becomes congested, or the baby is consistently distressed. You can ease this discomfort by using percussion, massage and a suitable decongestant oil on the chest area (see pp. 90–92)

3 weeks – 3 months

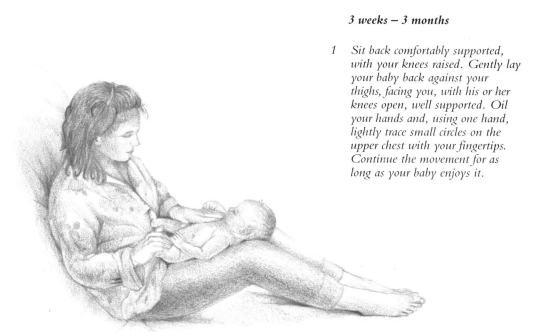

1   *Sit back comfortably supported, with your knees raised. Gently lay your baby back against your thighs, facing you, with his or her knees open, well supported. Oil your hands and, using one hand, lightly trace small circles on the upper chest with your fingertips. Continue the movement for as long as your baby enjoys it.*

2 Your baby may now relax his or
her arms, allowing you to extend
the movement. If this happens,
place your fingertips on the upper
chest. Lightly stroke upward and
outward across this area, out to
the shoulders and back again,
in broad circles. Repeat four or
five times.

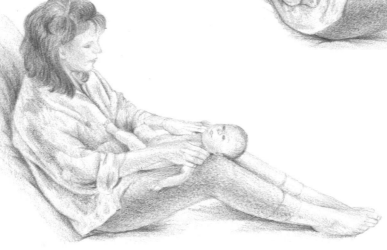

3 With your hands resting on
your baby's shoulders, use your
thumbs to stroke gently from the
centre of the breastbone outward,
making circular movements. At
the same time, lightly squeeze
the shoulders. Repeat, stopping if
your baby gets restless.

3 months onward

4 Sit back comfortably, on or
between your feet, and lay
your baby across your thighs,
on his or her back. Gently
support the head with one hand
as you lightly massage the upper
chest with your fingertips, using
circular movements. Gradually
extend the movement until first
your fingers, then your whole
hand, are touching the upper
chest. Continue for as long as it
is pleasurable.

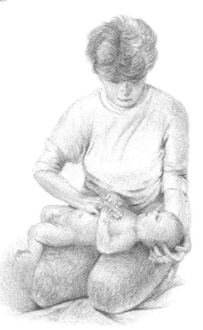

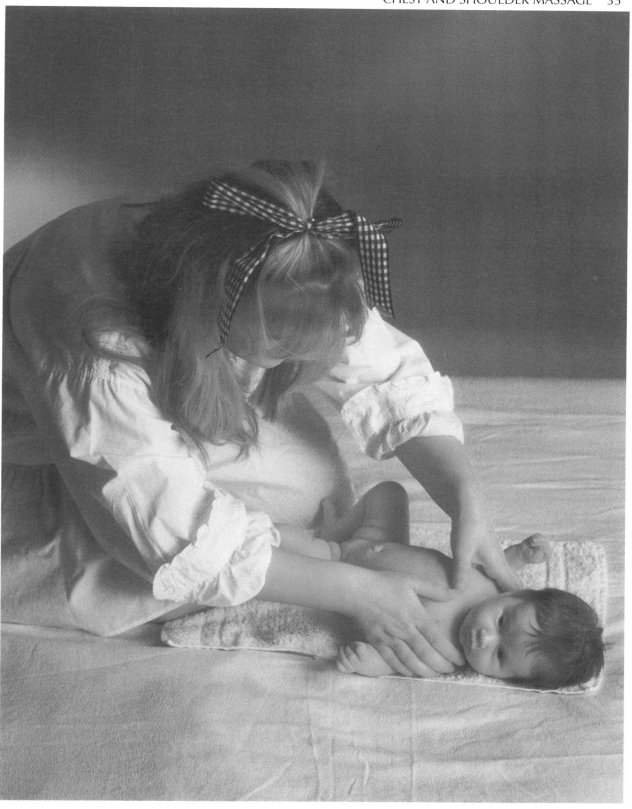

5 *Sit comfortably supported with your legs outstretched and apart. Sit your baby between your thighs, and let him or her lie back over one leg, while gently supporting the head with one hand. With the other hand, massage your baby's upper chest, as you did in step 4.*

6 *Bring your legs together and gently lay your baby along them, facing you, lifting your knees slightly. Softly place your hands over your baby's shoulders, and let your thumbs meet at the centre of the breastbone. Make light circular movements around the upper chest with your thumbs, at the same time squeezing the shoulders gently and drawing your hands out over the upper arms.*

7 *Sit back on your heels or between your feet, with your baby lying back comfortably on your lap, legs open around your waist. Gently rest the heels of your hands on the chest and tap lightly with your fingertips all around the upper chest. Talk to your baby as you do this, encouraging him or her to make sounds. This makes your baby aware of his or her voice resonating.*

ARM AND SHOULDER MASSAGE

Even before birth a baby begins to strengthen and co-ordinate the head and neck and arms and shoulders, and from birth onward, he or she continues to strengthen them in a variety of ways. If startled, very young babies will throw open their arms and draw them in again as if attempting to embrace one of their parents, and when lying tummy-down they will often lift and turn their heads. Lying on the tummy enables the baby to push upward and this strengthens the arms and shoulders. Naturally, you should let your baby lie in whatever position he or she finds most comfortable, but babies who find lying on the tummy uncomfortable often enjoy it more if a cushion is placed under their head and chest. Initially newborn babies hold their arms close to their bodies and their early movements are inclined to be a bit jerky. Given regularly, arm and shoulder massage will encourage re-laxation and co-ordination, and as the baby strengthens, will help to cultivate suppleness and flexibility in the major muscles and joints.

3 weeks – 3 months

1 *Sit with your back supported, knees raised, and gently lay your baby tummy-down over your thighs. Starting with your hands on the shoulders, glide them lightly down the upper arms, bringing the arms in to the sides of the body. Continue to glide your hands down over the elbows and rotate the lower arms gently inward so that your baby's palms turn in. Only continue the latter movement if your baby lets you - never force it.*

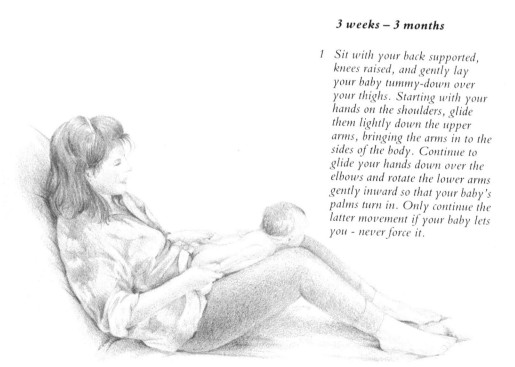

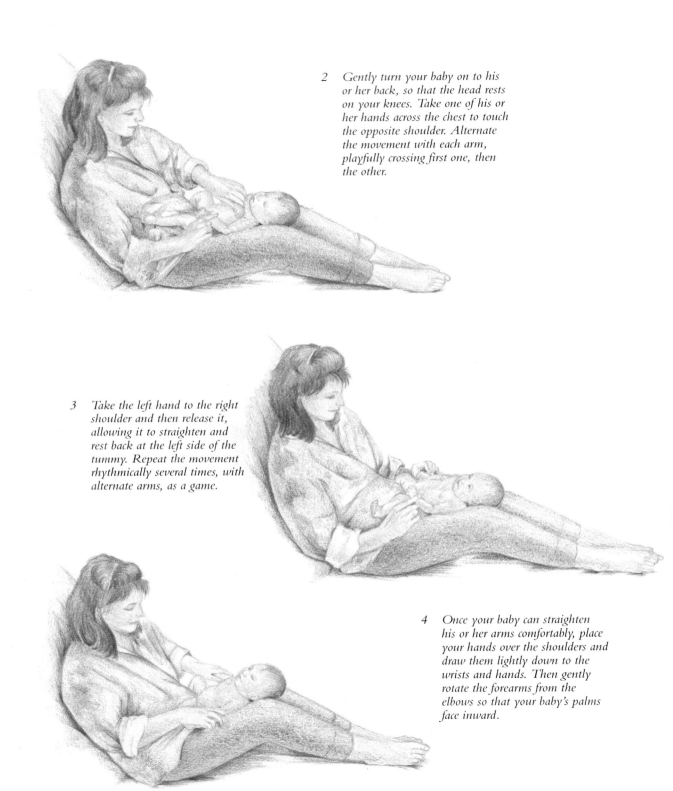

2   Gently turn your baby on to his or her back, so that the head rests on your knees. Take one of his or her hands across the chest to touch the opposite shoulder. Alternate the movement with each arm, playfully crossing first one, then the other.

3   Take the left hand to the right shoulder and then release it, allowing it to straighten and rest back at the left side of the tummy. Repeat the movement rhythmically several times, with alternate arms, as a game.

4   Once your baby can straighten his or her arms comfortably, place your hands over the shoulders and draw them lightly down to the wrists and hands. Then gently rotate the forearms from the elbows so that your baby's palms face inward.

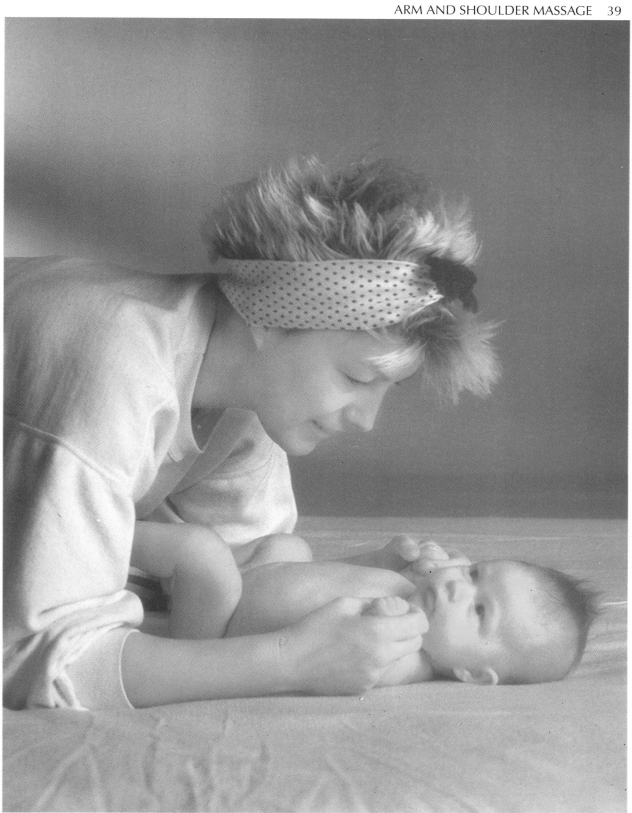

3 months onward

5 Sitting comfortably cross-legged, sit your baby down facing you. Then, **holding the forearms**, gently lift him or her into a standing position. Let your baby support some weight on his or her feet. Keep the arms outstretched, in line with the shoulders, and hold the position **only momentarily**. Repeat, if your baby enjoys it.

6 Now sit back on or between your feet, with your baby on your lap, leaning against your tummy. Oiling your hands, encircle the upper arms and draw your hands down to the wrists, while you "hug" your baby's arms back around the sides of your body, taking care to be gentle, and without using force. Keep the arms in line with shoulders.

7 Ensuring that your baby is leaning comfortably against your tummy, hold the forearms and lift them up gently, keeping the arms tucked into the body. Make sure the elbows are in line with the shoulders. Release, and repeat the movement, while talking and playing with your baby.

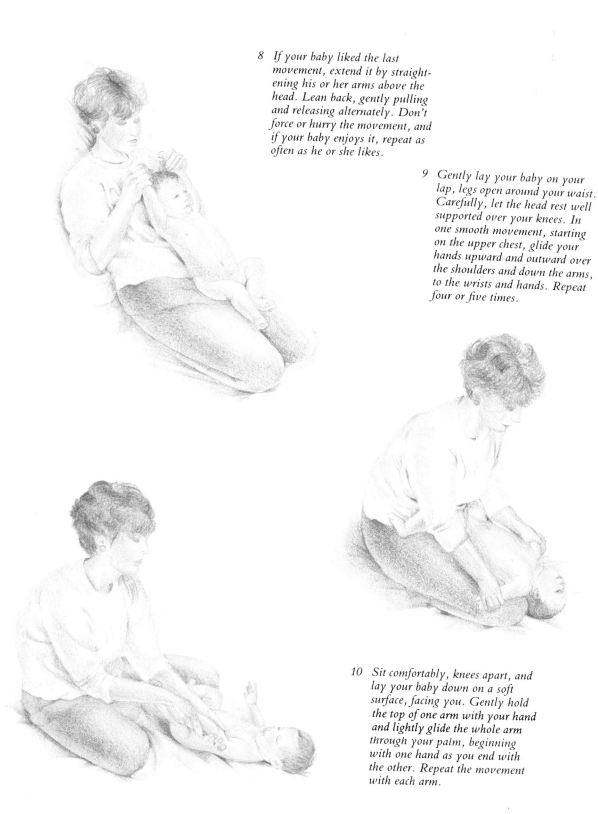

8 If your baby liked the last
movement, extend it by straight-
ening his or her arms above the
head. Lean back, gently pulling
and releasing alternately. Don't
force or hurry the movement, and
if your baby enjoys it, repeat as
often as he or she likes.

9 Gently lay your baby on your
lap, legs open around your waist.
Carefully, let the head rest well
supported over your knees. In
one smooth movement, starting
on the upper chest, glide your
hands upward and outward over
the shoulders and down the arms,
to the wrists and hands. Repeat
four or five times.

10 Sit comfortably, knees apart, and
lay your baby down on a soft
surface, facing you. Gently hold
the top of one arm with your hand
and lightly glide the whole arm
through your palm, beginning
with one hand as you end with
the other. Repeat the movement
with each arm.

TUMMY MASSAGE

For the unborn child the tummy is the centre of existence, the site of the umbilical connection with the mother that provides all that is needed to support life and growth. In the foetal position the tummy is not exposed as the body is curled around it. From birth, however, as the young baby begins to straighten the spine and limbs, he or she "opens" the front of the body and, contracting and strengthening, closes the back. Gently stroking your baby's tummy encourages the relaxation of the abdominal muscles and the general relaxation of the whole body, and this can also help to promote the digestive rhythm. When massaging the tummy, keep your touch light and pressure mininal and, as this is a very sensitive and vulnerable area, pay particular attention to your baby's responses. Some babies can ingest an uncomfortable amount of air when feeding and most often, traditional methods of burping or some light massage (with or without a suitable essential oil, see pp. 90–92) will bring relief. Gas, however, does not always account for a baby's distress, so don't overlook other possible causes – the root of the problem could be hunger, frustration, teething, illness, or simply the need for more physical reassurance.

3 weeks – 3 months

1   *Sit back comfortably supported knees slightly raised. Gently lay your baby down on your lap, facing you. Slowly open your baby's knees, letting the feet press against your tummy in a "squatting" position. Rock your baby playfully pushing first one knee, then the other, from side to side. Continue if your baby enjoys it.*

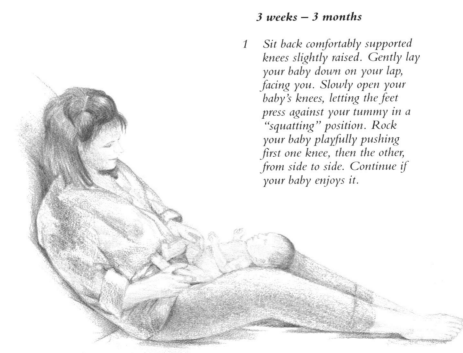

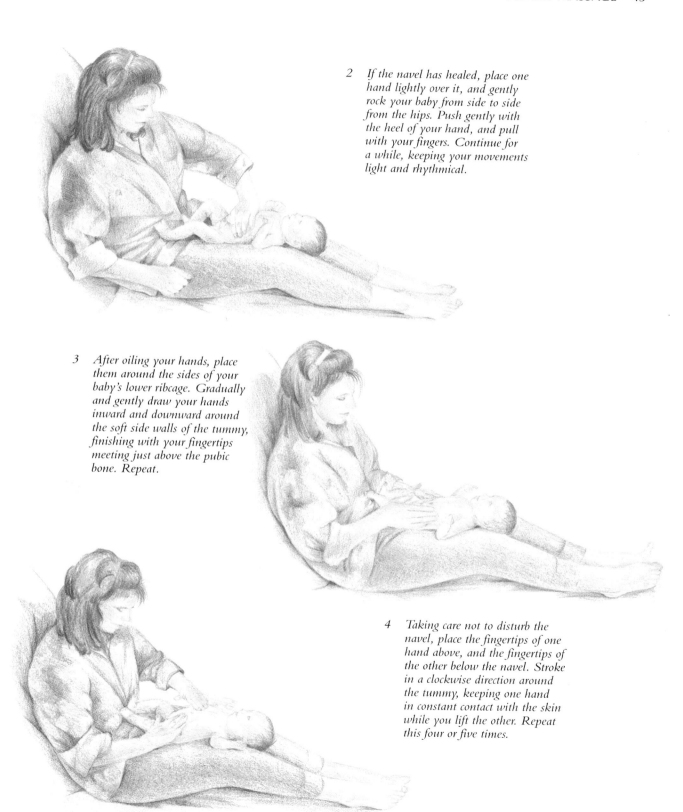

2   If the navel has healed, place one
    hand lightly over it, and gently
    rock your baby from side to side
    from the hips. Push gently with
    the heel of your hand, and pull
    with your fingers. Continue for
    a while, keeping your movements
    light and rhythmical.

3   After oiling your hands, place
    them around the sides of your
    baby's lower ribcage. Gradually
    and gently draw your hands
    inward and downward around
    the soft side walls of the tummy,
    finishing with your fingertips
    meeting just above the pubic
    bone. Repeat.

4   Taking care not to disturb the
    navel, place the fingertips of one
    hand above, and the fingertips of
    the other below the navel. Stroke
    in a clockwise direction around
    the tummy, keeping one hand
    in constant contact with the skin
    while you lift the other. Repeat
    this four or five times.

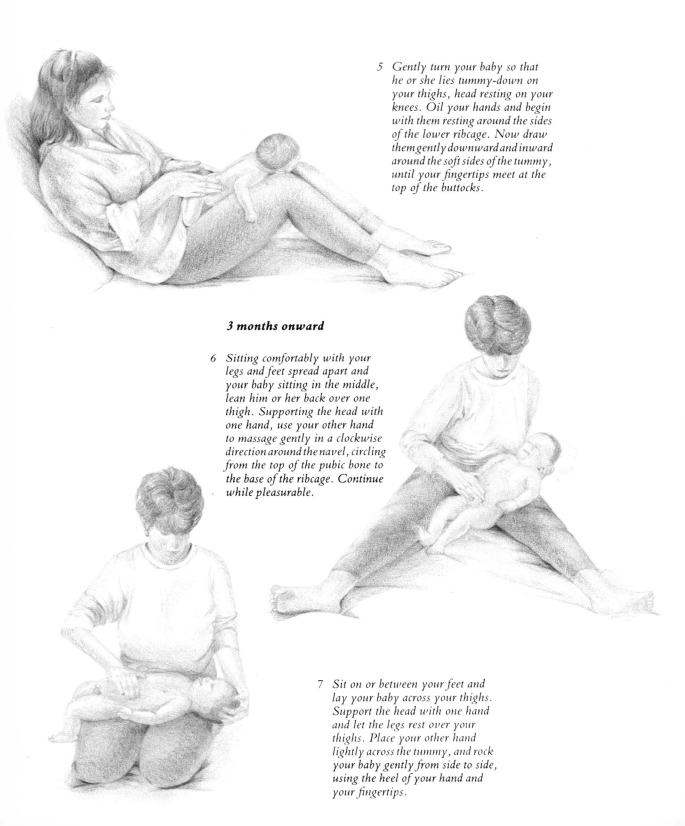

5 Gently turn your baby so that he or she lies tummy-down on your thighs, head resting on your knees. Oil your hands and begin with them resting around the sides of the lower ribcage. Now draw them gently downward and inward around the soft sides of the tummy, until your fingertips meet at the top of the buttocks.

3 months onward

6 Sitting comfortably with your legs and feet spread apart and your baby sitting in the middle, lean him or her back over one thigh. Supporting the head with one hand, use your other hand to massage gently in a clockwise direction around the navel, circling from the top of the pubic bone to the base of the ribcage. Continue while pleasurable.

7 Sit on or between your feet and lay your baby across your thighs. Support the head with one hand and let the legs rest over your thighs. Place your other hand lightly across the tummy, and rock your baby gently from side to side, using the heel of your hand and your fingertips.

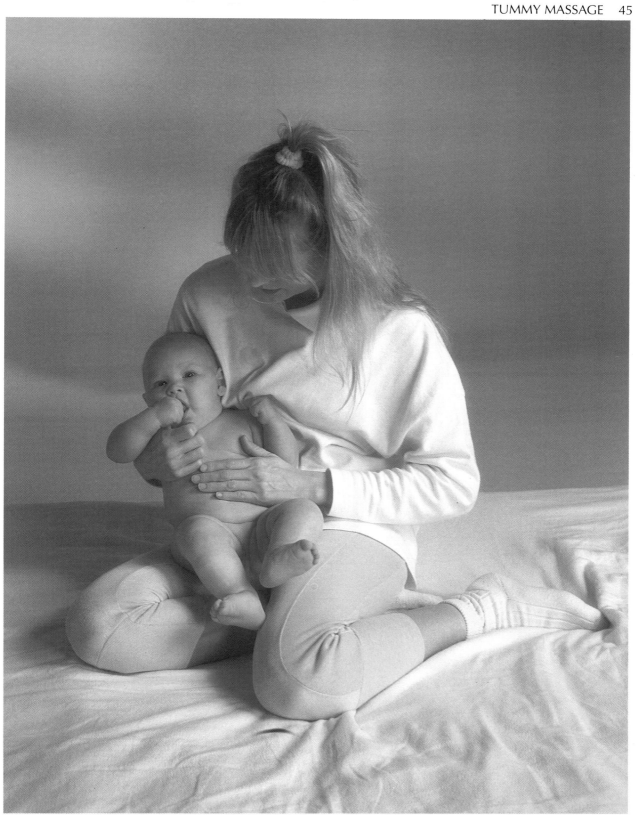

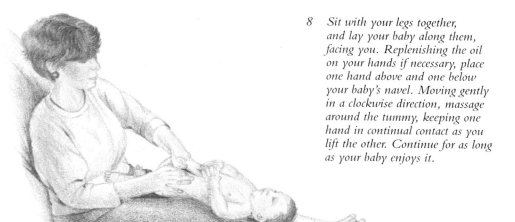

8　*Sit with your legs together, and lay your baby along them, facing you. Replenishing the oil on your hands if necessary, place one hand above and one below your baby's navel. Moving gently in a clockwise direction, massage around the tummy, keeping one hand in continual contact as you lift the other. Continue for as long as your baby enjoys it.*

9　*Sit on or between your feet, comfortably supported. Lay your baby down on your lap, facing you, legs open around your waist, head supported over your knees. In this position, massage the tummy in the same way as you did in step 8.*

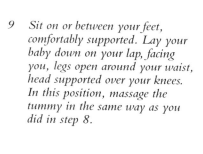

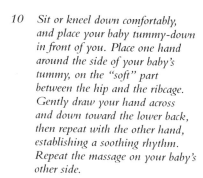

10　*Sit or kneel down comfortably, and place your baby tummy-down in front of you. Place one hand around the side of your baby's tummy, on the "soft" part between the hip and the ribcage. Gently draw your hand across and down toward the lower back, then repeat with the other hand, establishing a soothing rhythm. Repeat the massage on your baby's other side.*

BACK MASSAGE

The spine, the central pillar of support for the upper body, the central nervous system, heart, lungs, and digestive organs, is held erect through the strength of the back muscles. At birth, a baby has little strength in these muscles and the spine remains curled from the foetal position adopted in the womb. During the first months, through an intuitive pattern of movement, the young baby strengthens his or her back muscles and straightens the spine in preparation for upright postures and movements. The baby does this mainly by lying on his or her tummy and, by pushing with the arms and hands, arching his or her back and lifting the chest off the floor. Later you may see your baby lifting the head, chest, arms and legs simultaneously, a position that demands great physical strength and flexibility, well beyond the capabilities of the normal adult. Having strengthened the back muscles in this way from the head and neck downward the young baby is almost ready to sit upright. Massaging your baby's back muscles can be both soothing and stimulating. Depending on the pressure of your touch it encourages all the benefits of relaxation, co-ordination, and strength.

3 weeks – 3 months

1   *Lie back comfortably against a pile of cushions, legs extended. Carefully lay your baby on your chest, facing you. Oil your hands well and begin to massage the upper back gently with one hand, making clockwise circles.*

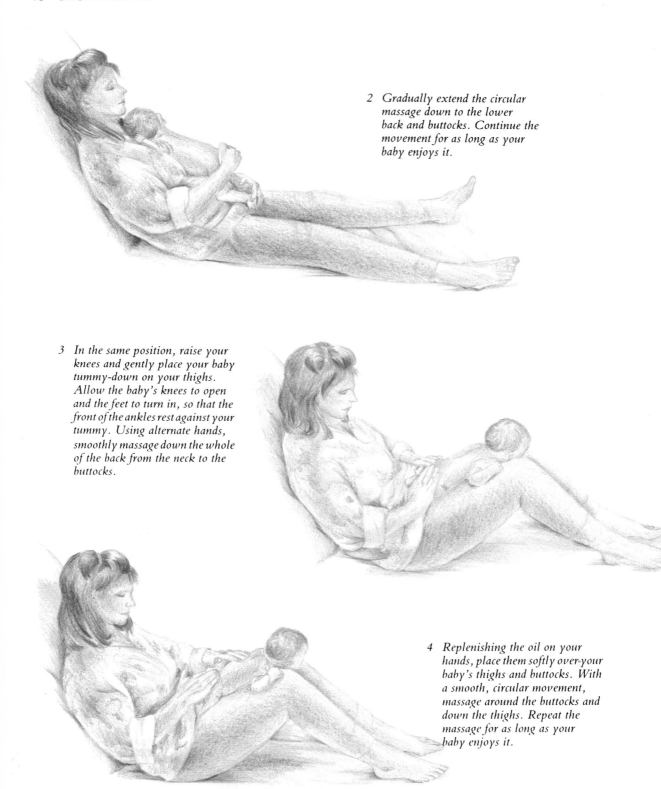

2 Gradually extend the circular
massage down to the lower
back and buttocks. Continue the
movement for as long as your
baby enjoys it.

3 In the same position, raise your
knees and gently place your baby
tummy-down on your thighs.
Allow the baby's knees to open
and the feet to turn in, so that the
front of the ankles rest against your
tummy. Using alternate hands,
smoothly massage down the whole
of the back from the neck to the
buttocks.

4 Replenishing the oil on your
hands, place them softly over your
baby's thighs and buttocks. With
a smooth, circular movement,
massage around the buttocks and
down the thighs. Repeat the
massage for as long as your
baby enjoys it.

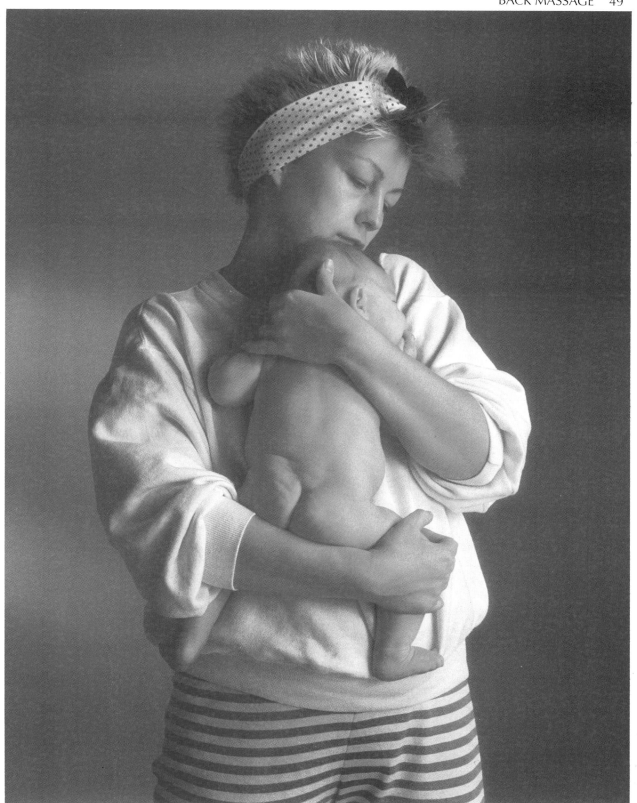

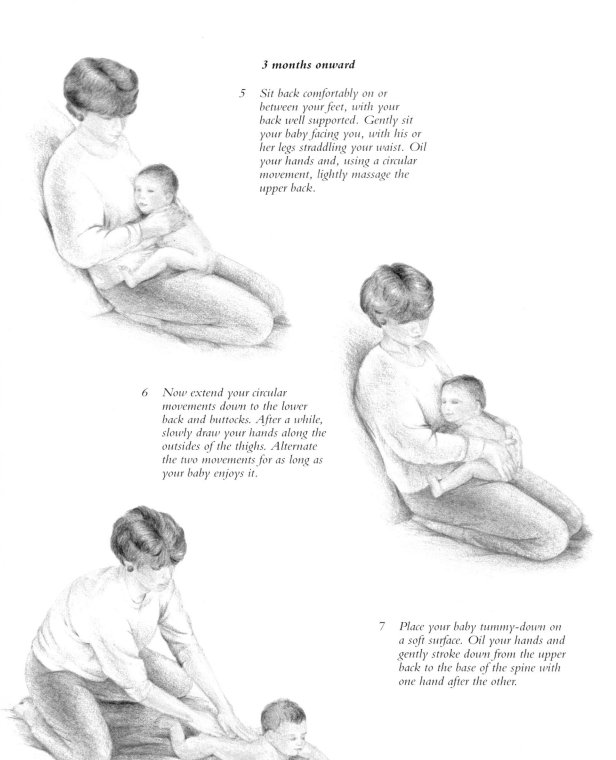

3 months onward

5   Sit back comfortably on or between your feet, with your back well supported. Gently sit your baby facing you, with his or her legs straddling your waist. Oil your hands and, using a circular movement, lightly massage the upper back.

6   Now extend your circular movements down to the lower back and buttocks. After a while, slowly draw your hands along the outsides of the thighs. Alternate the two movements for as long as your baby enjoys it.

7   Place your baby tummy-down on a soft surface. Oil your hands and gently stroke down from the upper back to the base of the spine with one hand after the other.

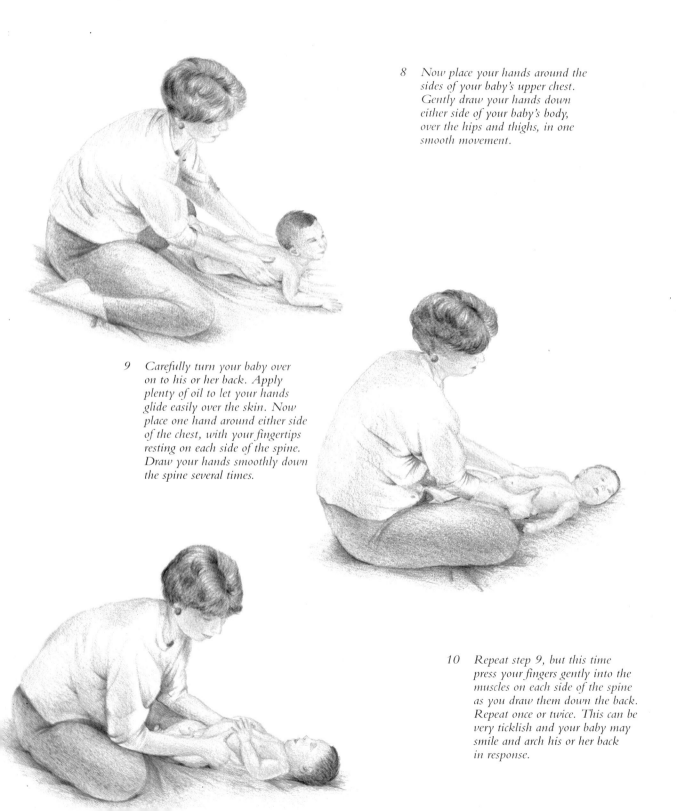

8   Now place your hands around the
     sides of your baby's upper chest.
     Gently draw your hands down
     either side of your baby's body,
     over the hips and thighs, in one
     smooth movement.

9   Carefully turn your baby over
     on to his or her back. Apply
     plenty of oil to let your hands
     glide easily over the skin. Now
     place one hand around either side
     of the chest, with your fingertips
     resting on each side of the spine.
     Draw your hands smoothly down
     the spine several times.

10   Repeat step 9, but this time
     press your fingers gently into the
     muscles on each side of the spine
     as you draw them down the back.
     Repeat once or twice. This can be
     very ticklish and your baby may
     smile and arch his or her back
     in response.

LEG MASSAGE

A baby's muscles strengthen and co-ordinate from the head and neck downward, so the legs are the last to strengthen and co-ordinate fully. From sucking their toes to standing with their heads touching the floor, as babies develop they display a wide range of extremely versatile movements that are well beyond the reach of most adults. Flexibility of the hip, knee, and ankle joints combined with suppleness in the postural muscles, the calves, thighs, and buttocks, make all these movements possible. The newborn baby holds his or her legs tucked into the front of the body and like any other part of the body, the legs should never be forcibly straightened, as the baby will straighten them in his or her own time. When massaging, bathing, or changing your baby, let the knees bend outward when the legs are extended toward the baby's face. Massaging the calves, thighs and buttock muscles encourages elasticity and co-ordination and keeps the legs flexible, all essential qualities for developing a good posture.

3 weeks – 3 months

1   *Lean back comfortably with your legs outstretched, knees raised slightly, and lay your baby on your lap, facing you, ensuring that the head and neck are well supported on your knees. Lightly hold the lower legs and gently press the knees inward toward the tummy. As soon as your baby begins to push back, facilitate the movement, and let the knees straighten — without pulling them. Repeat a few times.*

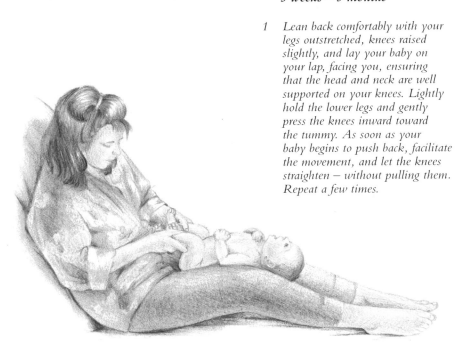

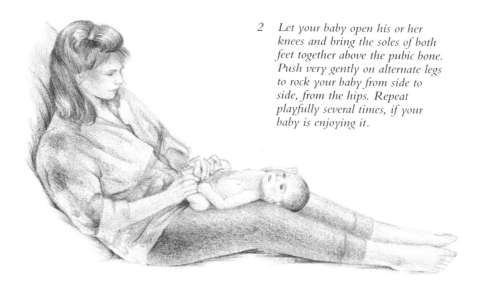

2   Let your baby open his or her knees and bring the soles of both feet together above the pubic bone. Push very gently on alternate legs to rock your baby from side to side, from the hips. Repeat playfully several times, if your baby is enjoying it.

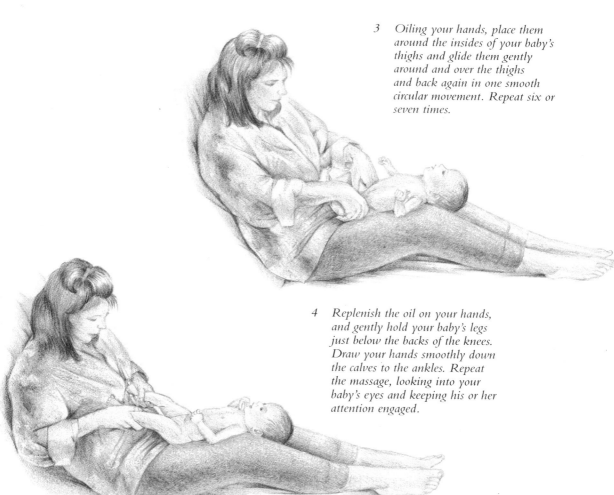

3   Oiling your hands, place them around the insides of your baby's thighs and glide them gently around and over the thighs and back again in one smooth circular movement. Repeat six or seven times.

4   Replenish the oil on your hands, and gently hold your baby's legs just below the backs of the knees. Draw your hands smoothly down the calves to the ankles. Repeat the massage, looking into your baby's eyes and keeping his or her attention engaged.

3 months onward

5   Sit back comfortably on or between your feet, or cross-legged, and place your baby on a soft surface, facing you. Gradually bring the soles of the feet together above the lower belly with one hand, and allow the knees to open. If comfortable, hold the position and massage around the buttock and down the back of the thigh with your other hand. Change hands and repeat on the other side.

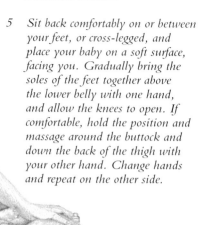

6   Lay your baby on his or her tummy. Gently press the instep of one foot to the buttock. If this is comfortable, hold the foot in this position and massage around the knee and down the front of the leg to the ankle. Repeat for both legs.

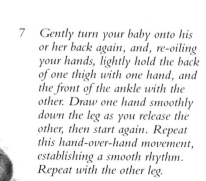

7   Gently turn your baby onto his or her back again, and, re-oiling your hands, lightly hold the back of one thigh with one hand, and the front of the ankle with the other. Draw one hand smoothly down the leg as you release the other, then start again. Repeat this hand-over-hand movement, establishing a smooth rhythm. Repeat with the other leg.

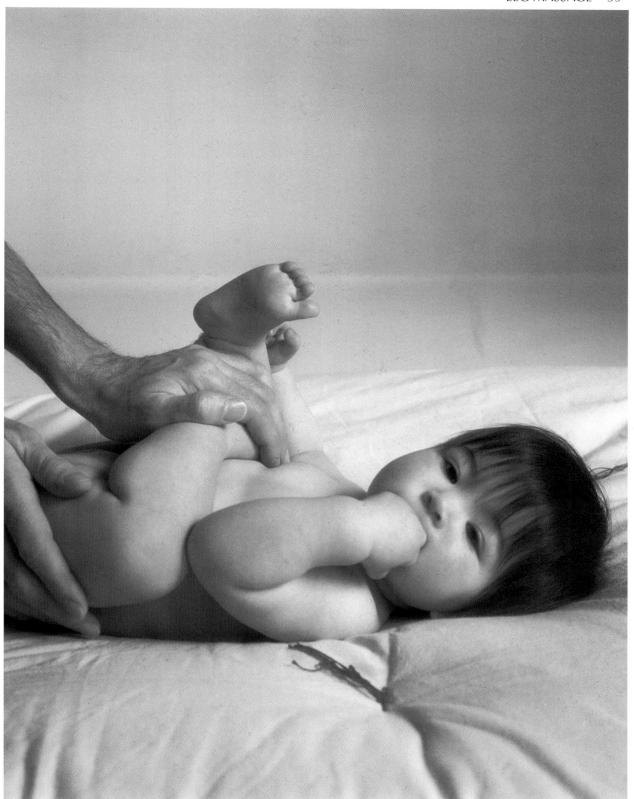

FACE AND HEAD MASSAGE

Your baby's face and head are very sensitive, and because the head is still growing there is usually a gap left for growth between the bones on top of the skull. Known as the fontanel, this is covered by a tough membrane and can be gently washed and touched. Most babies enjoy having their heads stroked and many find this soothing even when they are distressed. One of the most magical moments of parenthood is the baby's first smile, a moment of mutual happiness and recognition, and from this time on the baby's face begins to reflect his or her emotions. It is not unusual for a baby to dislike having his or her face stroked, however, so massaging the face should be approached with care and sensitivity, during those times that your baby is at his or her most receptive. Don't use oils, powders, or soaps on your baby's face because they can irritate delicate areas like the eyes and nasal membranes. The technique for opening the nostrils (see p. 58) is useful for relieving a blocked nose, especially when combined with a suitable decongestant oil (see pp. 90–92), but this is not meant to be a substitute for professional care.

3 weeks onward

1   *Sit or kneel comfortably with your baby lying on a soft surface facing you. Gently place your hand across the top of your baby's brow…*

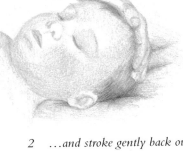

2   *…and stroke gently back over the head. If your baby is very young and the fontanel or "soft spot" has not closed, be extra careful when stroking around the top of the head. Repeat. This movement can be especially soothing for your child during fevers, teething, and other moments of distress.*

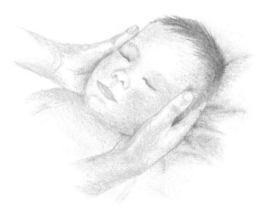

3   Place your relaxed hand around
    each side of your baby's head,
    with your thumbs on each side of
    the brow . . .

4   . . . and stroke gently outward with
    your thumbs, across the sides of the
    brow and over the hairline. Repeat
    six or seven times, keeping your
    movements smooth.

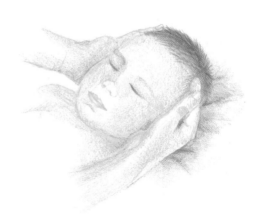

5   Now place your whole hands
    around the sides of your child's
    face, moulding your thumbs gently
    into the soft contours around the
    cheeks and cheekbones.

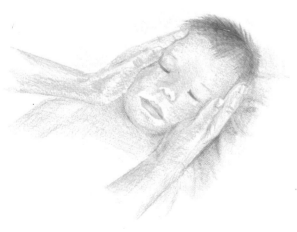

6   *Stroking lightly, draw your hands backward and upward, with the lower part of your thumbs, opening the cheeks and face gently. Repeat four or five times.*

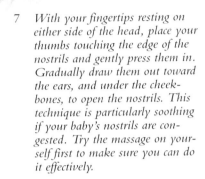

7   *With your fingertips resting on either side of the head, place your thumbs touching the edge of the nostrils and gently press them in. Gradually draw them out toward the ears, and under the cheekbones, to open the nostrils. This technique is particularly soothing if your baby's nostrils are congested. Try the massage on yourself first to make sure you can do it effectively.*

8   *With your fingertips in the same position, place your thumbs together under the mouth, just above the "jut" of the jawbone. Press in gently and draw your thumbs lightly outward around the jawbone. Repeat three or four times.*

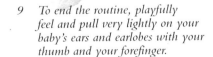

9   *To end the routine, playfully feel and pull very lightly on your baby's ears and earlobes with your thumb and your forefinger.*

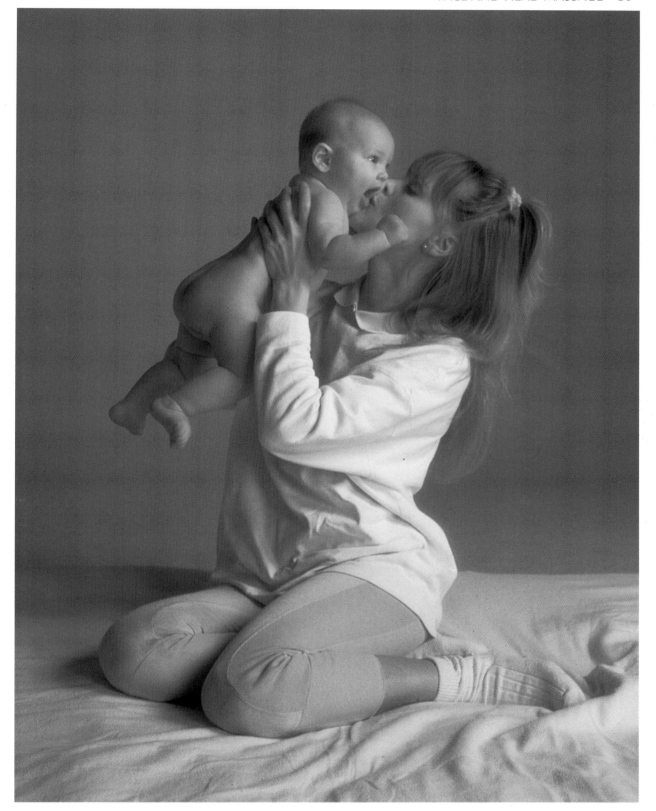

WHOLE BODY ROUTINE
3 weeks – 3 months

During this early period of development most babies graduate from sleeping through much of the day in the first few weeks to an average of three or four sleep periods at about three months. As your baby's need for sleep lessens, his or her need for more physical dialogue and social activity increases. "Body talk" – the name given to the physical communication that takes place between parent and child – cultivates a more expressive relationship, love, trust, and co-operation. To develop this and help fulfil your young baby's need for bodily contact and stimulation, introduce the following routine playfully and gradually. Check carefully what you need to know about oils and environment before you begin, then start by spending a few minutes on one part of the body. As your confidence grows include the entire body, one step at a time. The complete routine should take about twenty to thirty minutes, but can take as little or as long a period of time as you wish. Remember to talk, sing and keep your baby's attention fully engaged throughout, and be sure to remain attentive to your baby's responses.

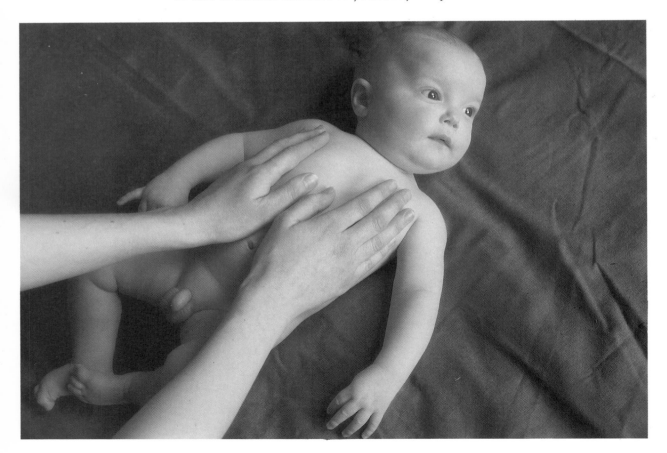

1   Place your baby on a soft surface, facing you. Relax your hands, oil them thoroughly, and place them gently over your baby's shoulders. Resting your thumbs on the centre of the breastbone, lightly stroke across the top of the chest, making opposing circles, or a figure of eight, with each thumb. Repeat the movement four or five times.

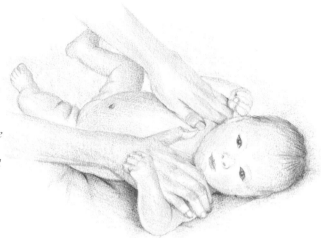

2   Slowly draw your hands across the tops of the shoulders and down the upper arms. Squeeze the upper arms gently. If your baby enjoys this, start from the beginning again, with your thumbs resting on the breastbone. This time draw your thumbs to your fingers and then glide your whole hands lightly over the shoulders and upper arms. Repeat for as long as your baby likes, talking and singing to your baby.

3   Hold your baby's forearms in the palms of your hands and slowly rotate the palms of your baby's hands inward as you gently straighten them downward along the sides of the body. Repeat as a game, four or five times. If your baby resists, leave it and try again later.

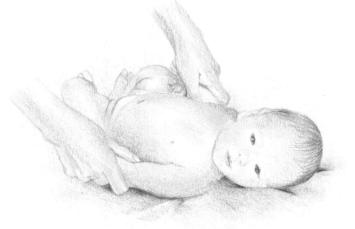

4   *When your baby is happy with this movement draw his or her forearms lightly through your palms four or five times. Then begin the whole sequence again from step 1, starting at the chest, and stroking over the shoulders and down the arms in one smooth movement. Repeat, guided by your baby's responses. This sequence encourages relaxation and co-ordination of the arms and shoulders.*

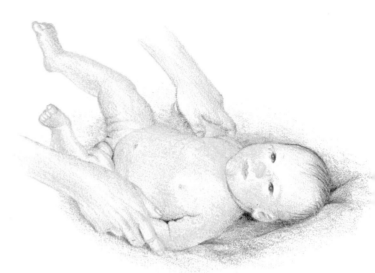

5   *Now place your hands around the sides of your baby's lower ribcage and draw them downward and inward, pressing gently into the soft side walls of the tummy. Let your fingertips meet above the pubic bone. Repeat four or five times, taking care not to disturb the navel if it has not yet healed.*

6   *Using the pads of your fingertips, place one hand above and one below the navel. Now moving in a clockwise direction — the same direction as your baby's digestive rhythm — stroke gently around the navel. Slowly widen the circle to include the entire tummy, keeping one hand in continual contact while lifting the other. Repeat as often as is enjoyable for your baby.*

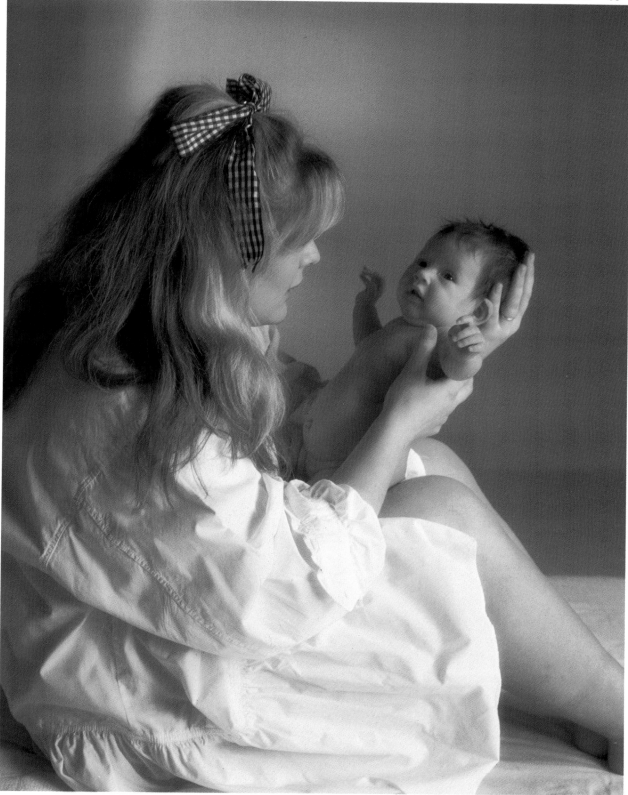

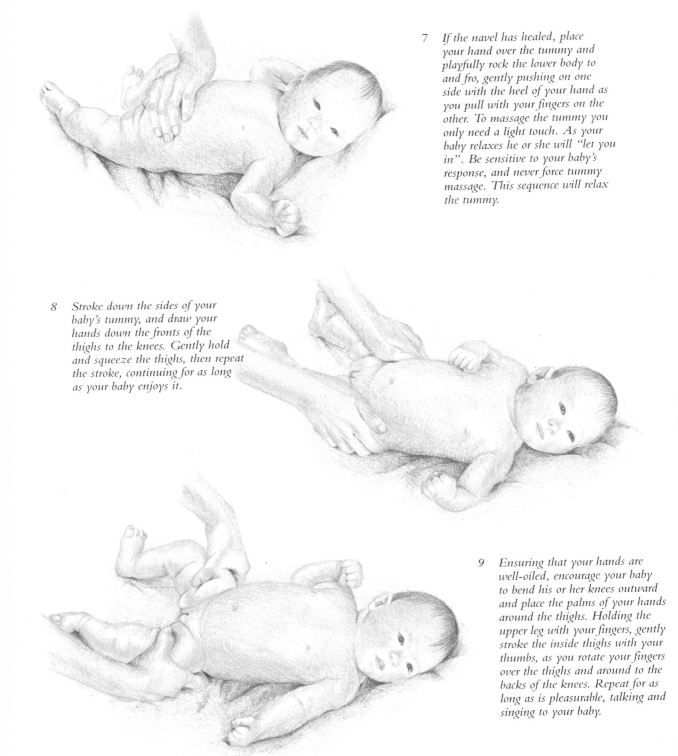

7   *If the navel has healed, place
your hand over the tummy and
playfully rock the lower body to
and fro, gently pushing on one
side with the heel of your hand as
you pull with your fingers on the
other. To massage the tummy you
only need a light touch. As your
baby relaxes he or she will "let you
in". Be sensitive to your baby's
response, and never force tummy
massage. This sequence will relax
the tummy.*

8   *Stroke down the sides of your
baby's tummy, and draw your
hands down the fronts of the
thighs to the knees. Gently hold
and squeeze the thighs, then repeat
the stroke, continuing for as long
as your baby enjoys it.*

9   *Ensuring that your hands are
well-oiled, encourage your baby
to bend his or her knees outward
and place the palms of your hands
around the thighs. Holding the
upper leg with your fingers, gently
stroke the inside thighs with your
thumbs, as you rotate your fingers
over the thighs and around to the
backs of the knees. Repeat for as
long as is pleasurable, talking and
singing to your baby.*

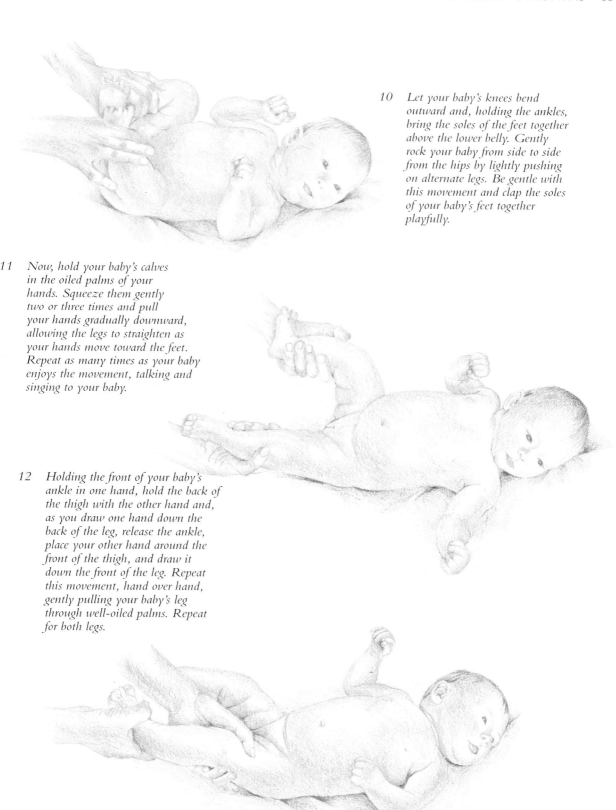

10   Let your baby's knees bend
outward and, holding the ankles,
bring the soles of the feet together
above the lower belly. Gently
rock your baby from side to side
from the hips by lightly pushing
on alternate legs. Be gentle with
this movement and clap the soles
of your baby's feet together
playfully.

11   Now, hold your baby's calves
in the oiled palms of your
hands. Squeeze them gently
two or three times and pull
your hands gradually downward,
allowing the legs to straighten as
your hands move toward the feet.
Repeat as many times as your baby
enjoys the movement, talking and
singing to your baby.

12   Holding the front of your baby's
ankle in one hand, hold the back of
the thigh with the other hand and,
as you draw one hand down the
back of the leg, release the ankle,
place your other hand around the
front of the thigh, and draw it
down the front of the leg. Repeat
this movement, hand over hand,
gently pulling your baby's leg
through well-oiled palms. Repeat
for both legs.

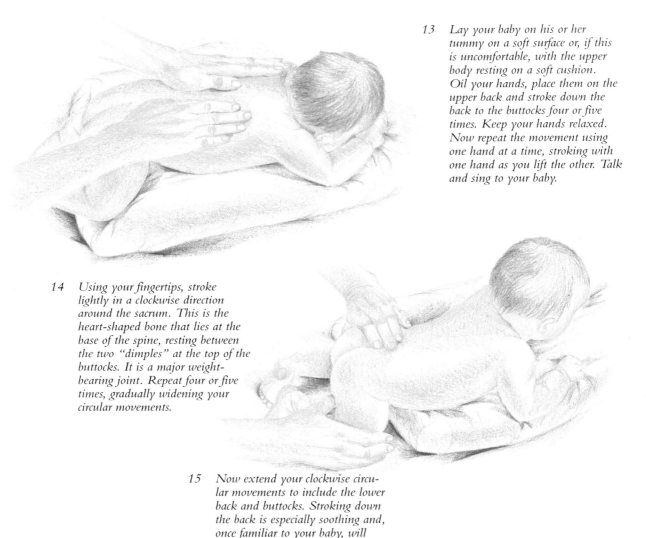

13   *Lay your baby on his or her tummy on a soft surface or, if this is uncomfortable, with the upper body resting on a soft cushion. Oil your hands, place them on the upper back and stroke down the back to the buttocks four or five times. Keep your hands relaxed. Now repeat the movement using one hand at a time, stroking with one hand as you lift the other. Talk and sing to your baby.*

14   *Using your fingertips, stroke lightly in a clockwise direction around the sacrum. This is the heart-shaped bone that lies at the base of the spine, resting between the two "dimples" at the top of the buttocks. It is a major weight-bearing joint. Repeat four or five times, gradually widening your circular movements.*

15   *Now extend your clockwise circular movements to include the lower back and buttocks. Stroking down the back is especially soothing and, once familiar to your baby, will have a very calming effect.*

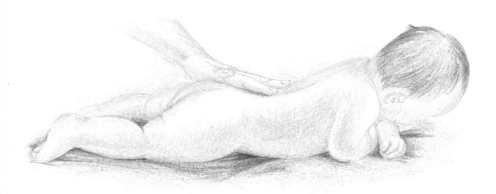

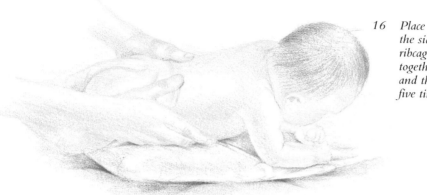

16   Place your relaxed hands around the sides of your baby's lower ribcage and draw them down together, stroking over the hips and thighs. Repeat four or five times.

17   Starting with your fingertips on your baby's buttocks glide your hands upward to cover them completely with the palms of your hands. Pressing very gently, massage both buttocks with both hands with circular movements. Then draw your hands down the tops of the legs.

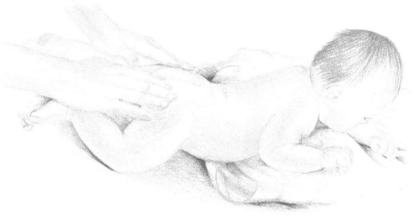

18   Now bend the right leg and gently press the right foot against the baby's buttocks. Afterwards, straighten the leg and stroke down from the hip to the foot. Then repeat for the left leg and foot.

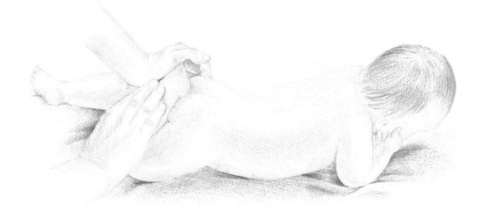

WHOLE BODY ROUTINE
From 3 months

From about three months, your baby is likely to be more active and to have developed greater strength and co-ordination – particularly in the head and neck, arms, shoulders, and upper back. At this stage, he or she may enjoy a slightly more energetic approach and a firmer touch on the less sensitive areas of the body. When you are both familiar with the following routine, therefore, try varying the rhythm and the pressure of your touch. Remain sensitive to your baby's responses, however, and continue to let your baby guide you. Before you begin make sure that you are relaxed and comfortable, and will remain so, and check that the room is warm enough. Talk and sing to your baby throughout, for if your attention begins to wander so will your baby's. The following routine is designed to complement your baby's development, to maintain suppleness and flexibility as your baby strengthens, to encourage co-ordination and relaxation and to promote proper functioning of the digestion, circulation and breathing. Above all, the routine is intended to give you the opportunity to develop a unique relationship, to touch and remain in touch with your baby.

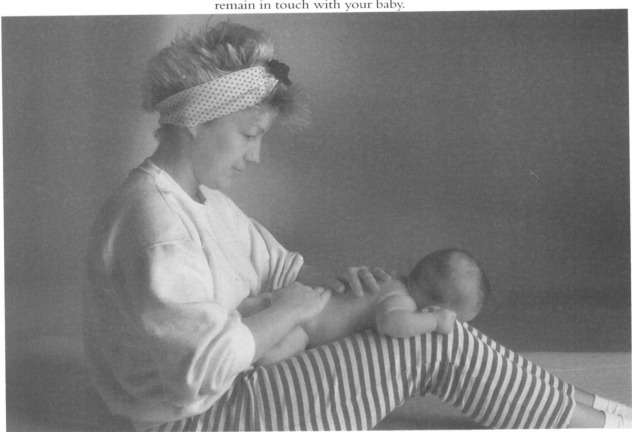

1   Place your baby on a soft surface, facing you, then oil your hands. Using the relaxed weight of your whole hands, stroke down the entire body from the shoulders, down the front of the chest and tummy, and down the legs and feet, to relax your baby. This does not necessarily include the genitals, but generally this area should be neither ignored nor accentuated.

2   Now place your hands on your baby's upper chest. Pressing lightly, glide your hands smoothly upward and outward over the chest and around the tops of the shoulders, then down the upper arms to the elbows. Keep your baby engaged as you repeat this about six times.

3   Ensuring that your hands are well-oiled, gently encircle the top of your baby's right arm with both hands. Pulling gently, glide hand over hand down the arm, letting go at the wrist with one hand as you begin at the top of the arm with the other hand. Repeat about six times with each arm, holding your baby's interest fully throughout.

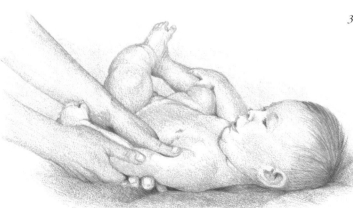

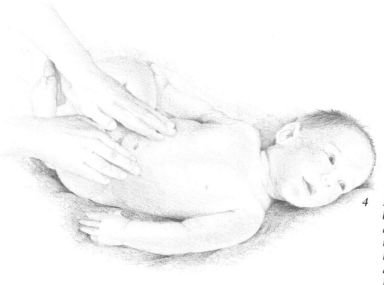

4   *Bring your hands back to your baby's chest and gently stroke down to the tummy three or four times. Now glide your fingers lightly in a clockwise direction around the navel, keeping one hand in continual contact with the skin, while you lift the other.*

5   *Now, using the relaxed weight of your hands, glide them in a clockwise direction around the navel, keeping one hand in continual contact and moving hand over hand. Include the entire tummy from below the ribcage to above the pubic bone. Maintain eye contact and talk or sing to your baby.*

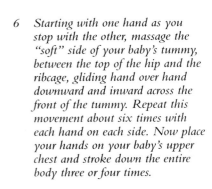

6   *Starting with one hand as you stop with the other, massage the "soft" side of your baby's tummy, between the top of the hip and the ribcage, gliding hand over hand downward and inward across the front of the tummy. Repeat this movement about six times with each hand on each side. Now place your hands on your baby's upper chest and stroke down the entire body three or four times.*

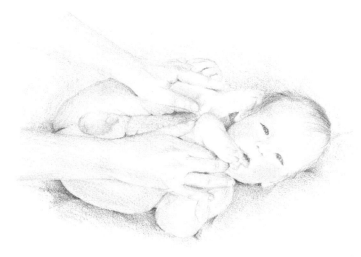

7   Gently hold your baby's ankles,
let the knees bend outward, and
bring the soles of both feet
together above the lower belly.
Now gently and playfully push
the feet toward the face, and allow
the lower back to lift. If your baby
resists, gently "clap" the soles
of the feet together. Don't force
the movement – let the baby's
responses be your guide. Talk and
sing to your baby.

8   Practising the same movements as
a gentle game, try rhythmically
pushing first one foot then the
other toward the face, allowing the
lower back to lift. Again, if your
baby resists, try clapping the soles
of the feet together, or kissing or
blowing on the feet. Otherwise,
leave it and try again when your
baby seems ready.

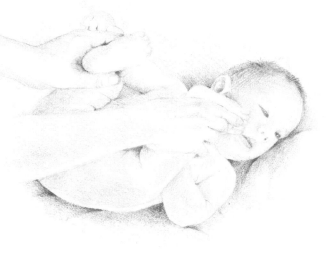

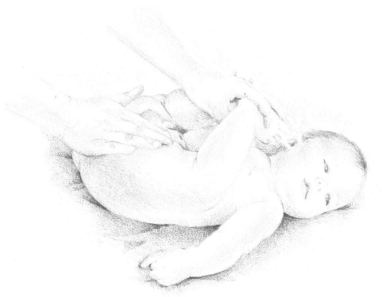

9   When your baby is comfortable
with movement 8, oil one hand
and gently hold both feet in front
of the face with the other one.
Place your oiled hand lightly on
the back of one thigh and glide
it in broad circles up toward the
knee joint and back, in a clockwise
direction . . .

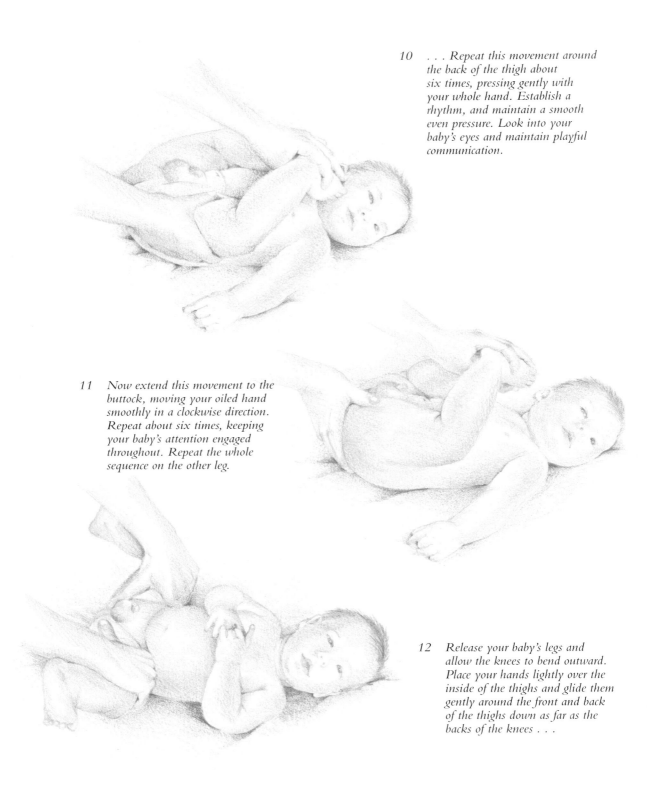

10   *. . . Repeat this movement around the back of the thigh about six times, pressing gently with your whole hand. Establish a rhythm, and maintain a smooth even pressure. Look into your baby's eyes and maintain playful communication.*

11   *Now extend this movement to the buttock, moving your oiled hand smoothly in a clockwise direction. Repeat about six times, keeping your baby's attention engaged throughout. Repeat the whole sequence on the other leg.*

12   *Release your baby's legs and allow the knees to bend outward. Place your hands lightly over the inside of the thighs and glide them gently around the front and back of the thighs down as far as the backs of the knees . . .*

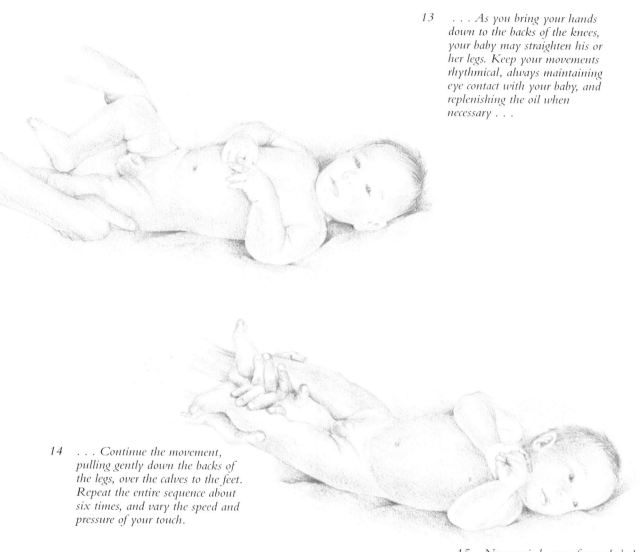

13   . . . As you bring your hands down to the backs of the knees, your baby may straighten his or her legs. Keep your movements rhythmical, always maintaining eye contact with your baby, and replenishing the oil when necessary . . .

14   . . . Continue the movement, pulling gently down the backs of the legs, over the calves to the feet. Repeat the entire sequence about six times, and vary the speed and pressure of your touch.

15   Now encircle one of your baby's ankles with one hand and gently hold the back of the thigh with the other. Slowly draw this hand down the back of the leg, release the ankle with the other one, and place it on the front of the thigh. Continue, gliding the leg through both your palms, hand over hand. Repeat with the other leg.

16   *Place your baby on his or her tummy on a soft surface, hands and arms extended forward. Using the relaxed weight of your hands, begin at your baby's shoulders and glide your hands down the back and legs to the feet. Repeat three or four times, kissing, talking, or singing to your baby.*

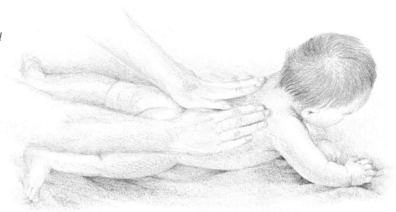

17   *Ensuring that your hands are well-oiled, place them over the backs of your baby's shoulders and draw them downward to the buttocks. Repeat this movement about six times, starting with one hand as you stop with the other.*

18   *To encourage the contraction and strength of these muscles — vital for your baby's upright posture and mobility — lightly tap or tickle your baby's back muscles on each side of the spine with your fingertips.*

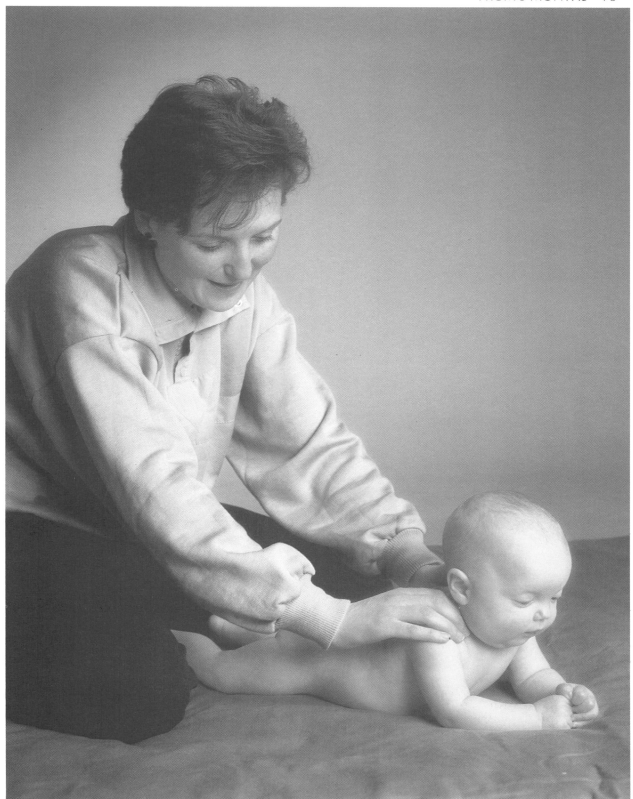

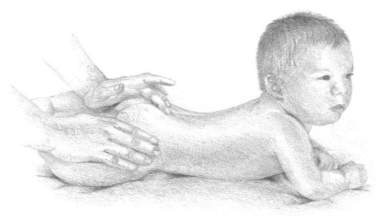

19   *Using just the fingertips, lightly massage around the sacrum, the heart-shaped bone at the base of the spine, in and above the fold in the buttocks. Repeat about a dozen times, engaging your baby's attention.*

20   *Now place both hands on the base of your baby's spine and glide them outward and around the buttocks in circular movements from the base of the spine. Continue for about six rotations, then draw your hands down the backs of the legs. Repeat about six times.*

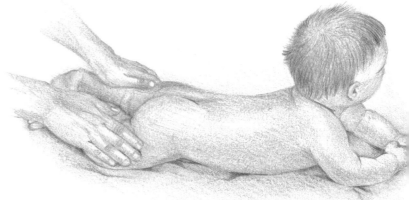

21   *Gently press the instep of each foot toward the buttocks and release. Repeat this movement two or three times and, if it is comfortable, press the instep of the foot gently to the buttocks and hold with one hand. Glide your other hand around the thigh and down the front of the lower leg. Repeat about six times.*

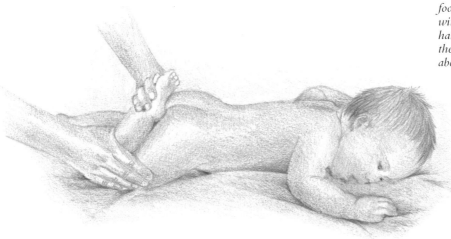

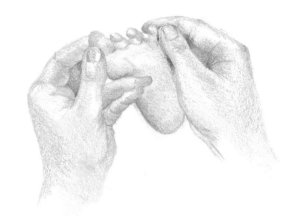

22   It's good to end by stimulating warmth and circulation in the hands and feet, as these extremities get cold most easily. Lay your baby down on his or her back and hold the large and the little toe with your forefingers and thumbs. Spread the toes, gently opening them like a fan…

23   …Taking the foot in both your hands, gently massage the sole with your thumb, and press around the base joint from where the toes emerge. Now take each toe and glide it through your thumb and forefinger, pulling gently. Repeat movements 22 and 23 as often as you and your baby enjoy them.

24   Now take one of your baby's hands and gradually open it, spreading the fingers like a fan. Press gently into the palm with your thumb and forefinger. Massage the joints at the base of the thumb and fingers. Massage both your baby's hands in this way.

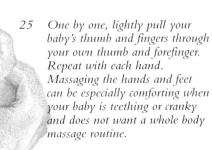

25   One by one, lightly pull your baby's thumb and fingers through your own thumb and forefinger. Repeat with each hand. Massaging the hands and feet can be especially comforting when your baby is teething or cranky and does not want a whole body massage routine.

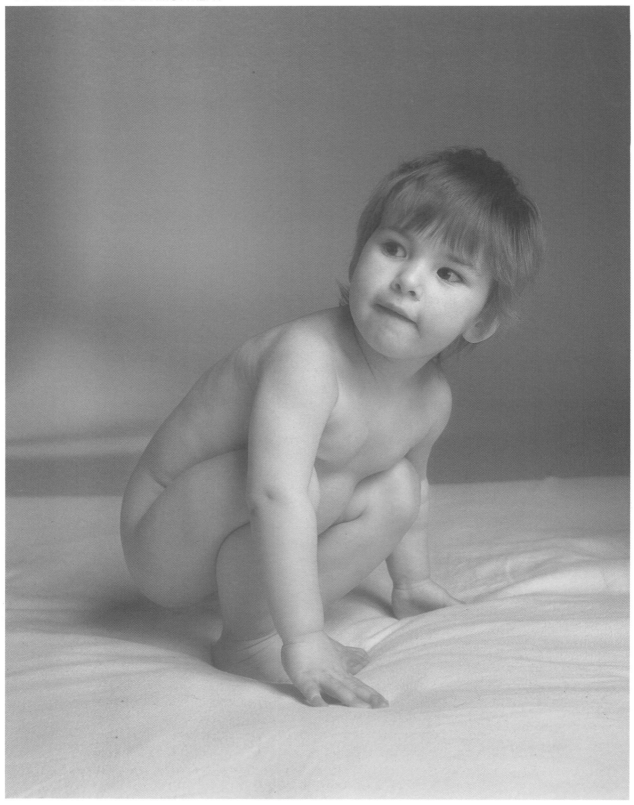

3

A BALANCED DEVELOPMENT

Babies the world over progress through the same sequence of stages of development – first sitting up, then crawling, standing, and taking the first steps. Every child develops these skills in much the same way, and is well rewarded for the effort by having more opportunity for social interaction and a greater degree of independence. The exact age when your child learns to sit, crawl, stand and walk is not important, however. Children vary greatly in their individual development patterns – some learn to sit early and walk late, while others sit late and walk early. As these motor skills demand the development and complex integration of your baby's muscles, bones, joints, and nervous system, they should never be hurried. But this does not mean that you cannot help your baby to prepare for these achievements.

In more "traditional" cultures than our own, children tend to develop their motor abilities far more quickly than their western contemporaries, because of the nature of their family relationships. These babies are held and carried almost constantly on their parents' bodies, and even when sleeping tend to remain in close physical contact with one or another member of their family. Fulfilling the baby's need for sustained physical contact establishes security and confidence. And this, combined with frequently holding the baby upright with the legs open astride the hips, allows him or her to develop the strength and flexibility needed for upright postures and mobility.

Both as a means of preparing the body for activity, and of relaxing it afterward, massage comes highly recommended by dancers, athletes, gymnasts, and others from all over the world. But at no time is it more beneficial than in early development, as your baby strives and prepares for upright postures and mobility. Once mobile, however, your baby is not likely to remain in one position long enough to engage in a complete massage routine, and he or she should not be pressurized into doing so. With a little gentle perseverance this can be easily changed in later infancy, but in the meantime your baby will still respond, during quieter, more restful moments, to massage given to receptive areas like the lower back and buttocks, and the upper back and head.

FROM LYING TO SITTING

Before beginning to crawl, your baby must first learn to sit upright, and this, in itself a major achievement, is usually accomplished between the fourth and the seventh month. In order to sit up, your baby needs to have developed strength and co-ordination in the muscles supporting the head and spine. And the hip joints need to be flexible as this allows the legs to open and provides a broad base on which to sit. Sitting upright also demands balance and this is achieved far more easily from a secure position. Rather than pulling your baby into a sitting position, you can help by sitting your baby upright, with the knees open and the feet together, and then leaning him or her forward on to a cushion. Like this, the baby is securely grounded and can use the arms and hands to push him or herself upright and then balance when ready. This position encourages your baby's arms, shoulders, and back muscles to strengthen and co-ordinate. When your baby can sit up unaided, he or she will be able to play a greater part in social activities – but don't leave your baby sitting alone until you are quite sure that he or she is perfectly safe and secure.

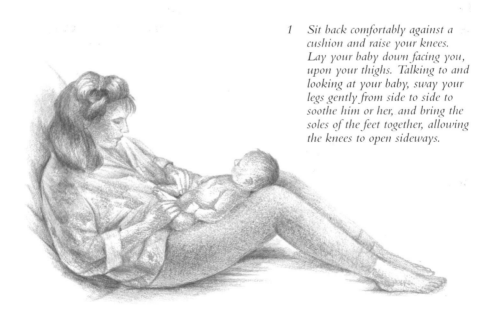

1   Sit back comfortably against a cushion and raise your knees. Lay your baby down facing you, upon your thighs. Talking to and looking at your baby, sway your legs gently from side to side to soothe him or her, and bring the soles of the feet together, allowing the knees to open sideways.

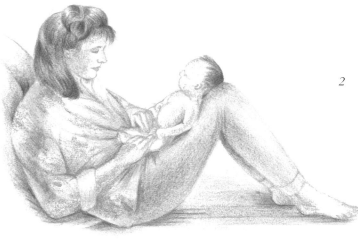

2   In the same position, slowly
raise your knees until your baby
is sitting more upright. Gently
sway your legs from side to side,
stroking the knees and lower
legs. This position encourages the
baby's legs to open and provide a
broad base on which to sit.

3   When you are sure your baby
has sufficient head control and
is comfortable in the previous
positions, sit back on your heels
with your knees open and sit your
baby between your knees, with
his or her back supported against
your tummy. Gently lift your
baby's arms over your thighs and
lightly stroke over the shoulders
and down the arms keeping your
movements smooth.

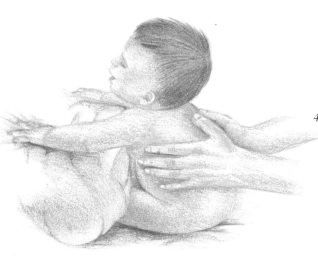

4   When your baby is familiar and
comfortable with position 3, sit
him or her in front of you, with
the feet together and the knees
open. Place a cushion over your
baby's legs and gently encourage
him or her to lean forward on to
the cushion. Lift your baby's arms
and gently extend them forward
over the cushion.

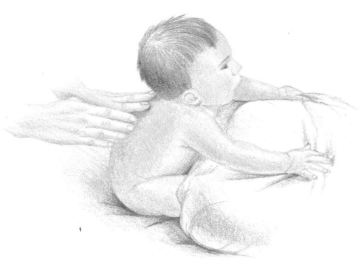

5   From this position your baby can push up into a proper sitting position and achieve balance in his or her own time. Encourage your baby by talking and singing to him or her and gently stroking the upper back in a circular movement with one hand. Also, stroke lightly down the back with both hands together. Don't leave your baby alone in this position.

6   When your baby can maintain position 5 comfortably for a few minutes at a time, take the cushion away. Hold your baby around both sides under the arms, and gently encourage your baby to support him or herself with the hands on the floor. Don't let your baby lean too far forward as he or she may become uncomfortable. Continue to practise this position with your baby until he or she can manage it unaided.

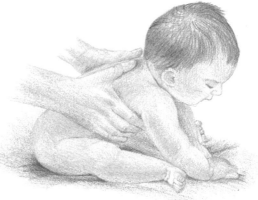

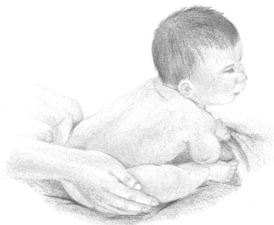

7   When your baby is comfortable in position 6, gently and carefully place your hands under his or her buttocks and pull them back to ensure that your baby is sitting on the backs of the legs and not on the buttocks. Gently stroke or massage down the back and around the buttocks and the sides of your baby's legs. Ensure that your baby is perfectly secure in this position before leaving him or her unsupervised.

FROM SITTING TO CRAWLING

Between about seven and twelve months, your baby will begin to develop mobility. Babies often pull themselves forward over their feet and on to all fours from a sitting position, and you can encourage this by placing toys in front of them once they are sitting securely. When on all fours babies are inclined to rock backward and forward and eventually find the second sitting position by sitting back between their feet. Some babies crawl on all fours, some shuffle along on their bottoms, while others pull themselves forward, trailing their legs and feet. To be able to crawl, a baby must strengthen and co-ordinate the legs and you can provide practical help by supporting your child in the right position as he or she "bounces" or squats and stands. Throughout this time your baby should continue to enjoy being massaged, but usually only on those parts of the body that are accessible without you needing to "position" him or her. Once mobile, the floor becomes your baby's domain and he or she will actively explore everything within reach. Rather than inhibit this natural curiosity and desire to investigate and learn, it is best to remove from the floor anything that is of value or potentially dangerous.

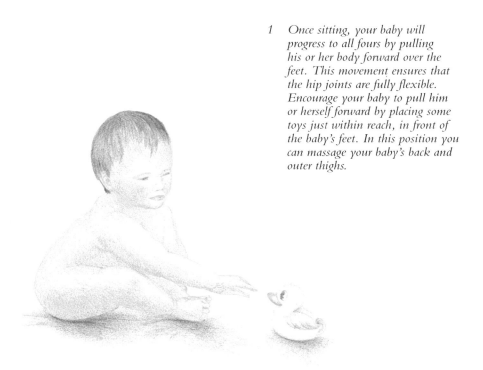

1   *Once sitting, your baby will progress to all fours by pulling his or her body forward over the feet. This movement ensures that the hip joints are fully flexible. Encourage your baby to pull him or herself forward by placing some toys just within reach, in front of the baby's feet. In this position you can massage your baby's back and outer thighs.*

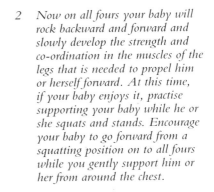

2   Now on all fours your baby will rock backward and forward and slowly develop the strength and co-ordination in the muscles of the legs that is needed to propel him or herself forward. At this time, if your baby enjoys it, practise supporting your baby while he or she squats and stands. Encourage your baby to go forward from a squatting position on to all fours while you gently support him or her from around the chest.

3   From all fours, your baby goes into the second sitting position, sitting back between the feet. This position encourages flexibility in the baby's knees and ankles. In this position massage your baby's shoulders, back, buttocks and legs.

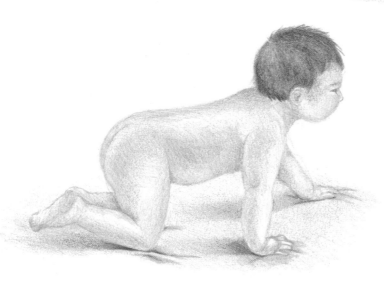

4   Once crawling, the whole floor becomes your baby's domain. At first, your baby will be far too busy exploring to remain still for massage. If you persevere during your baby's quieter moments, however, you will find that sooner or later he or she will respond to massage again.

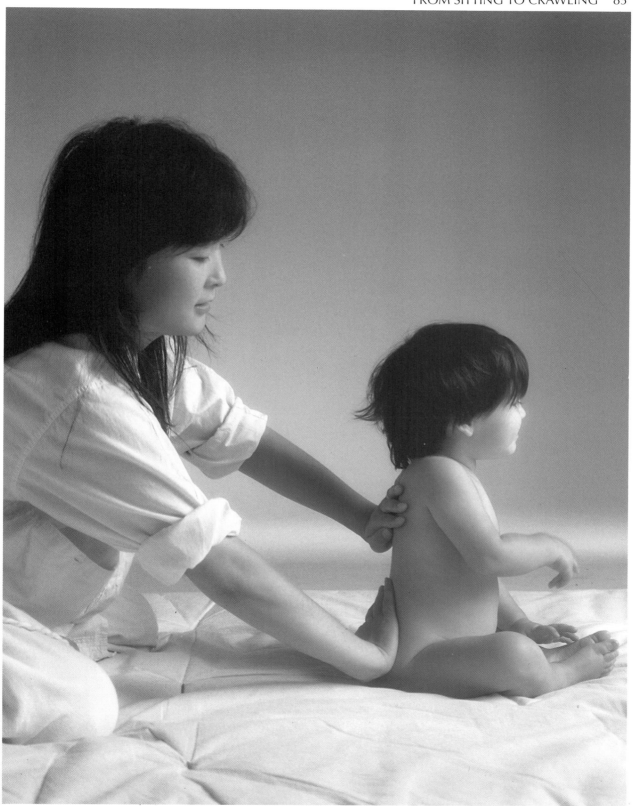

THE FIRST STEPS

Walking is an instinctive motor skill that forms the basis of much of our daily lives and recreational activities. From birth onward, babies held standing upright display an intuitive walking reflex and, though unable to support themselves, still seem to enjoy the feel of their feet on the ground. During the months that follow, as the baby gets stronger and gains more co-ordination from the head and neck downward, he or she can learn very gradually to support more and more weight when held standing. Once your child has developed good head control and the strength and co-ordination needed to support his or her back, you can begin to help by encouraging the first steps — a great adventure and achievement for your child. Holding your baby from the hips while he or she practises "bobbing up and down" will encourage the strength and co-ordination needed for sitting, standing, and walking unaided. Through trial and error and repeated effort your child will gradually strengthen and co-ordinate his or her legs and, in articulating these movements with others throughout the body, achieve balance.

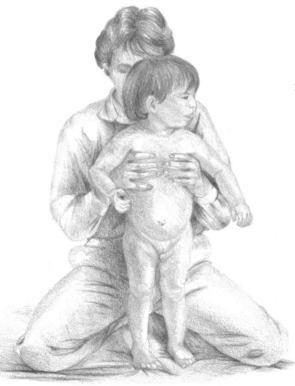

1   *Once your baby has achieved reasonable head control you can support him or her standing from under the arms. At first don't let your baby take too much of his or her weight on the feet for any length of time — just allow your child to feel his or her feet on the floor momentarily.*

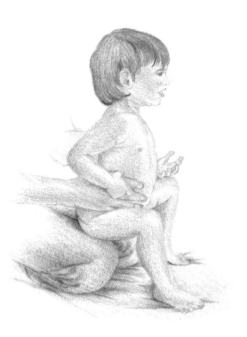

2   *Sit your baby astride one of your knees or, if you sit with straight legs open, astride your thigh. Hold your baby around the hips and if necessary, turn his or her feet to point in the same direction as the knees. This position will make it easy for you to support your baby for as long as it takes him or her to move from sitting to standing. You can practise this when your baby can support his or her head and back upright, even if he or she cannot yet sit unaided, as long as your baby enjoys it.*

3   *Standing upright from position 2 will help your baby to keep the legs and feet in line with each other and more open and will give him or her a broader base for balance. This position is best practised more consistently once your baby can sit unaided, as it will help to strengthen and co-ordinate the leg muscles for standing.*

4   *If your baby enjoys standing with your support, you can help him or her to achieve more balance by moving your hands downward. Support your baby from the hips and "bear down", gently pushing the legs and feet to the floor . . .*

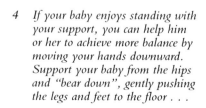

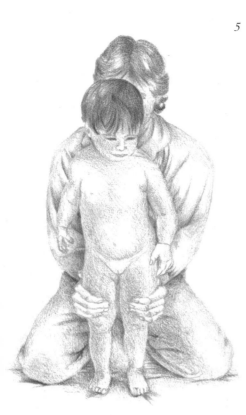

5   . . . *Now withdraw your support from the hips very gradually, by sliding your hands down the baby's legs, from the hips to the thighs to the knees. Do this very slowly, allowing your baby all the time that it takes to secure him or herself in one position before you move your hands down to the next. When supporting your baby from the legs, hold lightly and be ready to let go, as your baby will often step forward to secure his or her balance.*

6   Once your baby has developed a strong standing position, or can momentarily stand unaided, encourage walking by holding the hands from behind and letting him or her walk forward. In doing so let your baby take the lead and try not to hold him or her up by the hands. Instead, allow your child to pull or push on your hands when he or she feels the need for support.

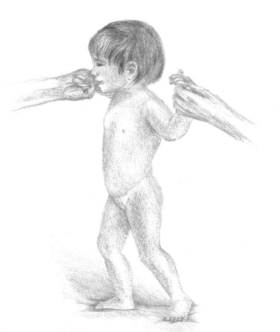

7   At about this time you may find your child pulling him or her-self up and walking with the aid of various pieces of furniture that are within reach of one another. When he or she is ready, encourage your baby to walk from you to your partner, letting go of one hand as your partner takes the other. In your baby's own time, slowly increase the distance between you and your partner.

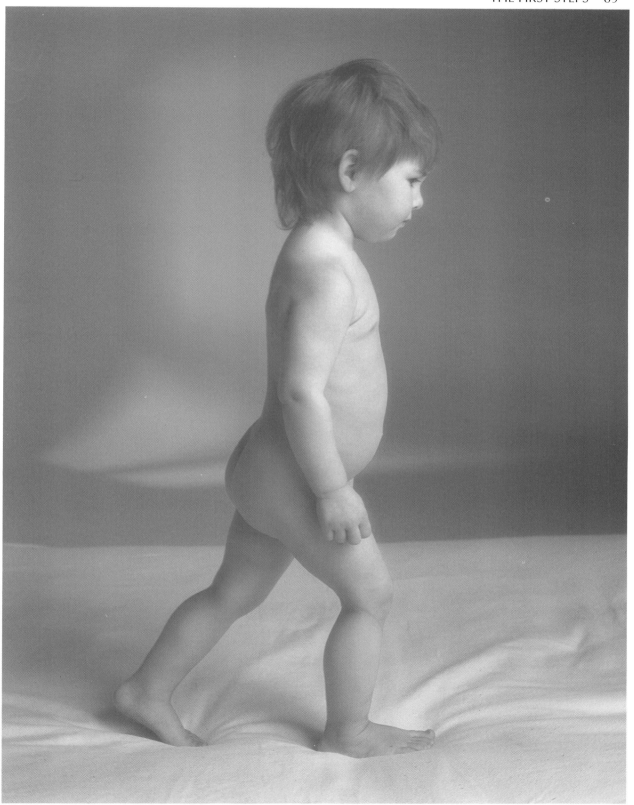

USING ESSENTIAL OILS
For minor ailments

As an aid to your baby's recovery from some minor ailments you can add a few drops of an essential oil to your basic massage oil and gently rub it in to the appropriate part of the body.

When using essential oils for massage you need to dilute them in an odorless oil, like grapeseed. For every one hundred milliliters of base oil, add twelve drops of essential oil or, for every two tablespoons of base oil, add three drops of essential oil. Always put a drop of diluted oil on a small area of your baby's skin first, and leave it for thirty minutes, to test for a reaction.

Camomile

A gentle oil with a calming and soothing effect, camomile is recommended for skin irritations and allergies. When gently massaged into the tummy, it is recommended to aid digestion, and when lightly rubbed into the cheeks (away from the eyes), it helps to relieve the distress of teething. Of the three kinds of camomile oil available, maroc, roman, and blue, camomile roman is the most suitable for use on a baby's skin, as it is non-toxic.

Lavender

This oil is most notable for its healing properties, which are enhanced by blending it with a base oil. It is recommended for soothing and healing minor burns and bites, but when using it for this purpose, on a small area of the skin, make a higher concentration with, say, forty per cent lavender to sixty per cent base oil.

Eucalyptus

This is a well-known and widely used decongestant. Massaged gently into your baby's back and chest before bedtime, it can be a great aid to a reasonable night's sleep in the event of a cough or a cold. Putting a little spot on your baby's pillow, or one on each side of the bed, can also help aid restful sleep.

Myrtle

Myrtle belongs to the same family as eucalyptus, and has the same properties.

Peppermint

Cooling and soothing, peppermint also has decongestant properties. It is recommended for relieving the discomfort of gas if you massage it very lightly into your baby's tummy.

Rose

Although rather expensive, rose has excellent all-round restorative properties. Associated with love and the heart, the oil of the rose is emotionally soothing; it benefits and softens the skin and is non-toxic.

Benzoin

This is a gum resin, non-toxic, with an aroma like vanilla. Like rose, it is associated with the heart. The oil is warming and, when massaged into your baby's chest or back, eases the discomforts of a cough or cold.

Frankincense

The oil of frankincense has a low toxicity level and is deeply relaxing, with a pleasant aroma that deepens the breathing rhythm.

Myrrh

A resin similar to frankincense, myrrh is non-toxic and contains warming elements. It is recommended for soothing inflammations of the bronchial tubes and expelling mucus.

Teatree

Teatree is non-toxic and, despite its powerful antiseptic qualities, is a non-irritant. It is recommended for soothing and healing wounds and skin infections.

Note: Essential oils should not be used as a substitute for professional diagnosis and treatment. And they are for external use only – on no account should they be taken internally.

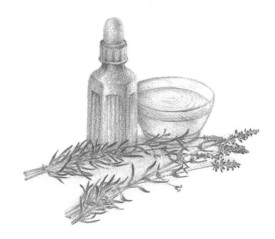

MASSAGE FOR MINOR AILMENTS

This chart provides a simple reference guide for you to use in conjunction with the recommendations on essential oils given on pages 90–91. For the common infant ailments or symptoms listed, apply the relevant essential oil, diluted with a base oil (see page 90), and combine it with the appropriate massage technique.

Note: Seek professional advice promptly, if symptoms persist.

Ailment	Massage	Essential oil
Skin irritations or allergies	massage gently into affected area	camomile, rose, teatree
Minor burns or bites	massage gently into affected area	lavender
Coughs or colds	"opening the nostrils" (p. 58) percussive massage on chest (pp. 23, 33)	eucalyptus, peppermint, benzoin, myrtle
Chest congestion	percussive massage on chest and back helps break down mucus (pp. 23, 33, 47)	eucalyptus, peppermint, myrrh, benzoin, myrtle
Digestive disorders	gentle tummy massage (pp. 42, 90)	camomile
Teething	stroking the cheeks (p. 90) massaging the hands and feet (p. 77)	camomile
Gas	very light tummy massage (p.42)	peppermint
Irritability or sleeplessness	In particular stroking down whole body (p. 69), gently stroking the tummy (p. 42) back massage (p. 47) and head massage (p. 56)	rose, frankincense

INDEX

RESOURCES

Recommended Reading

Brazelton, T. Berry, TOUCHPOINTS: YOUR CHILD'S EMOTIONAL AND BEHAVIORAL DEVELOPMENT, Addison-Wesley, 1994

Sears, William M. and Martha, THE BABY BOOK: EVERYTHING YOU NEED TO KNOW ABOUT YOUR BABY – FROM BIRTH TO AGE TWO, Little, Brown, 1993

Leach, Penelope, YOUR BABY & CHILD, Knopf, 1989

Zukow, Bud and Nancy Sayles Kaneshiro, BABY: AN OWNER'S MANUAL, Kensington, 1996

Clarke, Jean, ed., HELP! FOR PARENTS OF CHILDREN FROM BIRTH TO FIVE: TRIED-AND-TRUE SOLUTIONS TO PARENTS' EVERYDAY PROBLEMS, HarperCollins, 1993

Spock, Benjamin M. and Michael B. Rothenburg, DR. SPOCK'S BABY AND CHILD CARE, NAL-Dutton, 1992

Eisenberg, Arlene et al, WHAT TO EXPECT THE FIRST YEAR, Workman, 1988

Taubman, Bruce, WHY IS MY BABY CRYING?: THE SEVEN-MINUTE PROGRAM FOR SOOTHING THE FUSSY BABY, Simon & Schuster, 1993

Useful Addresses

Lamaze
American Society for Prophylaxis in Obstetrics (ASPO/Lamaze)
1200 19th Street NW, Suite 300
Washington, DC 20036-2401
202-857-1128
800-368-4404
Information and support for natural childbirth

American Academy of Husband-Coached Childbirth
Box 5224
Sherman Oaks, CA 91413-5224
800-4ABIRTH
Information on childbirth education; workshops and lists of instructors

New Parents' Network
P.O. Box 44226
Tucson, AZ 85733-4226
(520) 881-8474
Information on pregnancy and early childhood parenting

International Association of Infant Massage
1720 Willow Creek Circle
Suite 516
Eugene OR 97402
(800) 248-5432
Certification in infant massage; will supply list of local instructors

The General Touch Warehouse
1720 Willow Creek Circle
Suite 518
Eugene, OR 97402
(888) 448-9489
Massage related materials: literature, pure oils, instructional cassettes and videos

Pourquoi Pas, Inc.
1115 Liebau Road
Suite 200
Mequon, WI 53092
414-377-6722
800-422-2987
Distributor of massage oils and infant and childhood skin-care products

American Academy of Pediatrics
141 Northwest Point Boulevard
Elk Grove Village, IL 60067
(708) 228-5005
(800) 433-9016
Information on medicine, health and nutrition

La Leche League International
1400 North Meacham Road
Schaumburg, IL 60173
(847) 519-7730
(800) 525-3243
Information and support for breastfeeding

Parents Without Partners
401 North Michigan Avenue
Chicago, IL 60611
(312) 644-6610
(800) 637-7974
Information and support for single-parent families

Women's Legal Defense Fund
1875 Connecticut Avenue NW
Suite 710
Washington DC 20009
(202) 986-2600
Information and support on family issues

DANVILLE, INDIANA